Advanced Myofascial Techniques

Til Luchau

Volume 2

Neck, head, spine and ribs

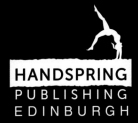

HANDSPRING
PUBLISHING
EDINBURGH

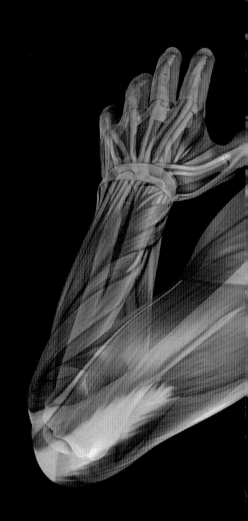

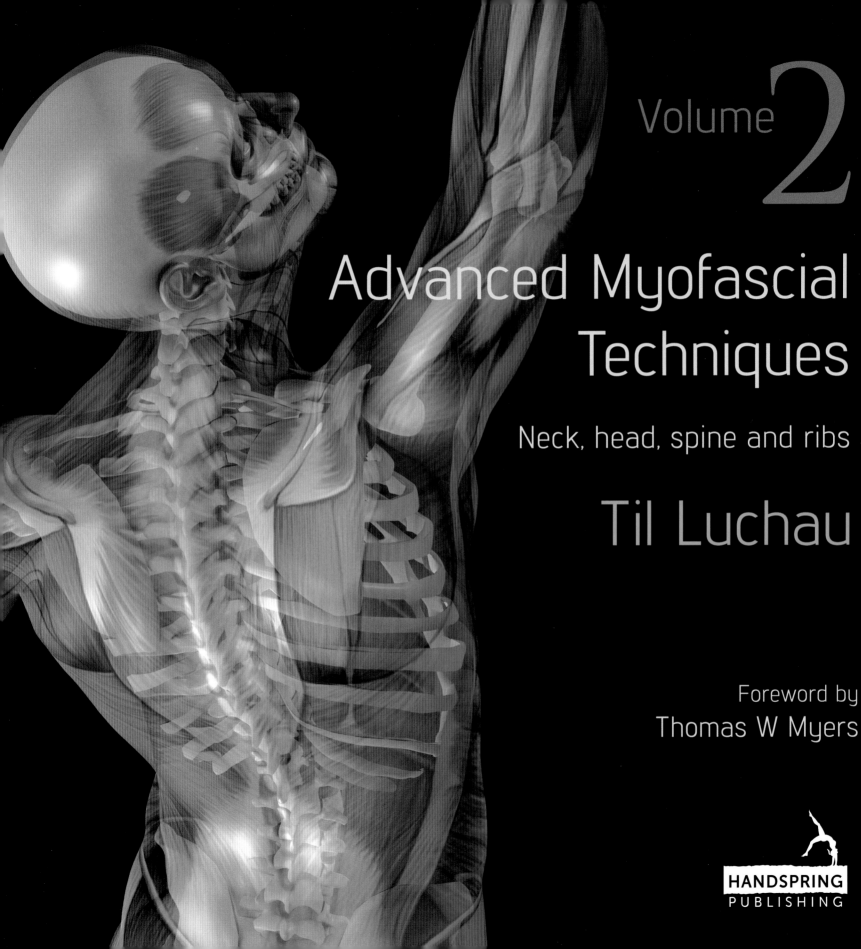

Volume 2

Advanced Myofascial Techniques

Neck, head, spine and ribs

Til Luchau

Foreword by
Thomas W Myers

HANDSPRING
PUBLISHING

HANDSPRING PUBLISHING LIMITED
The Old Manse, Fountainhall,
Pencaitland, East Lothian
EH34 5EY, Scotland
Tel: +44 1875 341 859
Website: www.handspringpublishing.com

First published 2016 in the United Kingdom by Handspring Publishing
Reprinted 2016
Reprinted 2017
Reprinted 2019
Copyright © Til Luchau 2016
Illustration copyrights as indicated at the end of each chapter

ISBN 978-1-909141-17-9

British Library Cataloguing in Publication Data
A catalogue record for this book is available from the British Library

Library of Congress Cataloguing in Publication Data
A catalog record for this book is available from the Library of Congress

Notice

Neither the Publisher nor the Author assumes any responsibility for any loss or injury and/or damage to persons or property arising out of or relating to any use of the material contained in this book. It is the responsibility of the treating practitioner, relying on independent expertise and knowledge of the patient, to determine the best treatment and method of application for the patient.

Commissioning Editor Sarena Wolfaard
Design direction and Cover design by Bruce Hogarth, KinesisCreative
Artwork by PrimalPictures unless otherwise indicated
Project Management by NPM Ltd
Index by Aptara
Typeset by DSM Soft
Printed in the Czech Republic by FINIDR

Contents

Contents

Headaches

Closure and Sequencing

Foreword

It is perhaps unfair to invoke the author's younger self when introducing a book from his later years, but I remember so vividly the impression Til Luchau made when first I met him more than 20 years ago. Whip-thin, with such an offhand air of quiet and calm surrounding his movements, his low and understated voice – it all suggested someone, one might infer from a first glance, not quite up to the energetic job of teaching for which he was auditioning.

A second look, however, into the probing assessment emanating from his clear green eyes was enough to reveal that the first laconic impression is merely a veneer, a gentle Gen X presentation covering for a fiercely inquiring and stubbornly thorough Renaissance mind. A mind willing to generously entertain the intuitions and inclusiveness of 'alternative' medicine, but unwilling to settle for complacent half-truths that too often take the place of the complex totality of clinical experience.

Also in his favor, following the example of Buckminster Fuller and John Lilly, Til has always used himself as his own scientific guinea pig, living out his questions into the answers so clearly presented here. From deep yoga practice to juggling devil sticks, Til has played with his own mind and body, constantly using himself to test the edges of flexibility and coordination, practicing the preparation, differentiation, and integration fractals so integral to mastering the processes described in this book.

Needless to say, Til was definitely up to the job of teaching, and I subsequently bequeathed the entire program to his competent hands. In the intervening years, his native skills have been further honed by continual and varietal practice. The detailed research underlying these volumes is testimony to his assembly and careful sifting over time of the evidence around the questions that surround contemporary manual therapy.

In this series, Til makes liberal and salient use of the un-traditional views of anatomy now available through electronic media, exposing relationships not evident in the standard texts. The photographs included not only show the techniques as they apply to the client, but also where the intent is directed vis-a-vis the client's skeleton - a boon to accurate application across different body types. Charts, summaries, and study guides only add to the clarity of the presentation for the mid-level or advanced manual therapist.

I am very happy to see that this second volume covers the vestibular system, which is sadly underserved elsewhere, as well as dealing openly and fairly with the controversies surrounding the psoas major and environs. Other corners at the edge of manual therapy's reach, such as the diaphragm, rib heads, mesentery and deeper structures of the neck are dealt with in a practical but sophisticated manner.

As Til states, a book is a good but limited tool, so augment the information from here with his video presentations, or enjoy the mature version of the unique man I saw so many years ago by going to Til's classes. You can rely on what you find, because his innate confidence is such that he feels no need to overstate his case or claim 'cures' or causation. The spirit of this book is exploration, an informed exploration that encourages the client's body to heal itself, and evokes the client's desire to retain the renewed access to movement.

And most of all, Til's work requires the practitioner to stay awake and aware, the single most important factor in a long and satisfying practice.

Thomas Myers
Author of *Anatomy Trains*
Clarks Cove, Maine
January 2016

Acknowledgements

The acknowledgements in this book's first volume thanked 37 people, and yet still didn't manage to include everyone who had helped that book's creation. Because these two volumes were written together, each of the people listed there should, by rights, be thanked once more.

Author, practitioner, and fascial researcher Robert Schleip PhD should again receive special mention for the inspiration, encouragement, and support he has so freely given to me, and to so many others in our field. Thomas Myers, Jan Sultan, Art Riggs, Erik Dalton, and many other mentors and colleagues have also lent invaluable and direct support.

Leslie Young PhD and Darren Buford hosted many of the first drafts of this material in *Massage & Bodywork* magazine, as did Anne Williams via ABMP's online webinar series.

I am deeply indebted to the many who generously gave permission or granted license to use their images. Primal Pictures deserves special mention. They are listed in each chapter's image credits, but all deserve a special thanks for sharing their vision and hard work.

Kate Dennington and Patrick Dorsey both worked especially hard on the first-draft versions of the study guide questions and key points, and helped make the work applicable to day-to-day practice. Advanced-Trainings.com faculty Bethany Ward, Larry Koliha, George Sullivan, Chris Pohowsky, and Ellyn Vandenberg all contributed important ideas, editing, dialog, and support, as did the international community of colleagues, teaching assistants, hosts, and students engaged in this work, such as Carmen Rivera in San Juan, Puerto Rico, Bibiana Badenes in Benicassim, Spain, Cheryl LoCicero in Edmonton Alberta, Canada, Simone Baianu in San Francisco, California, Jasmine Blue and East West College in Portland, Oregon, as well as many others.

I am most grateful to the many hospitable people who very graciously provided a few days or a few weeks of quiet writing-time refuge on my itinerant teaching circuit. Anna Maria Gregorini in Zurich; Wendy Hooker in Fairbanks; Poh Yap in London; Wojtek Cackowski in Poland;

Acknowledgements

Bruce Nelson in Anchorage; Budiman Minasney in Sydney; Finnbogi Gunnlaugsson in Reykjavik: all went above and beyond.

Special thanks to Andrew Stevenson, Sarena Wolfaard, Bruce Hogarth, and Katja Abbott at Handspring Publishing for their collaborative spirit.

And to my family Loretta Carridan Luchau and Ansel Luchau, for their understanding and heartwarming care.

Til Luchau
Boulder, Colorado, 2016

Introduction

This book continues the theme begun in Volume I of Advanced Myofascial Techniques (Handspring Publishing, 2015). In Volume I, you will find a discussion of essential background information about the goals of this style of work; the nature of the tissues we are affecting with this modality; and descriptions of a selection of hands-on techniques for conditions of the appendicular skeleton, specifically the upper and lower limbs, and the shoulder and pelvic girdles.

This second volume takes this discussion deeper, presenting manual therapy approaches for client complaints related to the axial skeleton: the spine, abdomen, ribcage, neck, and head; concludes with some considerations relevant to sequencing these techniques into sessions or a series of sessions.

The techniques in these volumes have been specially selected for their accessibility, relevance, and effectiveness, from amongst the more than 350 assessments, techniques, and procedures that constitute the curriculum of the ever-expanding Advanced Myofascial Techniques series of seminars and videos. This repertory of techniques has been clarified and refined over the course of more than 30 years of clinical practice, professional continuing education trainings, and practitioner supervision. They will be natural additions to a wide range of therapeutic, rehabilitative, and educational methods, including structural integration (to which they owe their primary inspiration), physical and physiotherapy, occupational therapy, massage therapy (both rehabilitative and restorative), chiropractic, osteopathic manipulation, craniosacral therapy, speech therapy, orthodontics, sports and conditioning training, movement therapy, yoga, and many other methodologies concerned with the health and functioning of the physical body.

Using this book

This book can be used on its own, or alongside the full Advanced Myofascial Techniques video series, or as a complement to the certification programs and in-person professional continuing education trainings of the same name.

Introduction

Whether you're using this book as a part of a systematic course of study, or meandering through it on your own, you will get the most out of it if you actually do the techniques. Don't wait until you've gone through the entire book to try them out. Even if you begin by just looking at the images, or watching a video link, put a friend or a colleague on the table as soon as you can, so that your hands and body can learn the material as you go through it. Once you've actually tried a technique, go back and take in another aspect of the material, perhaps reading the key point summaries, or the text, or reviewing the study guide questions and their online answer keys. When you work through the material in this way, you will learn the material more fully, and will have begun the process of making these techniques your own.

The techniques in these volumes can be incorporated one-by-one into your existing work and protocols, *à la carte* fashion, according to the indications and purposes listed in each technique's Key Points section, or as you see fit. If you're a big-picture learner, skip ahead to the final chapter, *Sequencing*, early in your reading. This will give you a context for the way these techniques can be organized into sequences, sessions, or series. If you prefer to just start working, go right ahead: dig into the techniques themselves, and visit Chapter 20 on sequencing when you're ready.

Together with Volume I, this book provides effective ways to work with some of the most common client complaints. It is designed to significantly expand your skillset and get you thinking differently about ways to help your clients. It is not intended to be a comprehensive pathology text, nor does it cover everything you need to know about the conditions discussed. As a book of techniques for professionals and advanced students, it is assumed that the reader has familiarity with the basic contraindications and cautions related to hands-on work, as well as in-person training in the sensitive application of pressure, and as well as the therapeutic relationship, bedside manner, the ethical and legal considerations related to hands-on work, etc.

Of course, no book, even with video supplementation like this one has, can take the place of live training. A book is no substitute for the real-time coaching and mentoring that occurs during an in-person course, nor can it replace the crucial experiential knowledge gained by receiving the work yourself—at a minimum, find a colleague or friend to work on you, so that you can experience the most important aspect of this approach—receiving it.

Til Luchau
Boulder, Colorado, 2016

Reviewers

Bibiana Badenes, P.T.
Physical Therapist, Certified Advanced Rolfer™, Certified Rolf Movement® Teacher; Director, Kinesis Center and Movement Therapy; President, BodyWisdom Foundation Spain
Benicàssim, Spain.

Erik Dalton, Ph.D.
Certified Advanced Rolfer™; Author;
Executive Director, Freedom From Pain Institute
Oklahoma City, Oklahoma, United States.

Rachel Fairweather BA, LMT, AOS Massage therapy, CQSW
Director, Jing Advanced Massage Training; Author
Brighton, United Kingdom.

Cheryl LoCicero, B.Sc. R.M.T
Certified Advanced Rolfer™, Certified Rolf Movement® Teacher, Fascial Integration: Structural-Visceral approaches
Consultant, Center for Complementary and Alternative Research and Education, University of Alberta
Edmonton, Alberta, Canada.

Budiman Minasny, Ph.D.
Researcher, University of Sydney
Sydney, Australia.

Peter B. Pruett, M.D.
Physician – Board Certified in Emergency Medicine
Delta County Memorial Hospital
United States Air Force Academy; University of Colorado, Denver
Hotchkiss, Colorado, United States.

Art Riggs
Certified Advanced Rolfer™; Author
Director, Art Riggs Deep Tissue and Manual Therapy Educational Systems
Berkeley, California, United States.

Susan G. Salvo, M.Ed., L.M.T.
Author – Educator – Massage Therapist
Louisiana Institute of Massage Therapy
Lake Charles, Louisiana, United States.

Robert Schleip, Ph.D. M.A.
Visiting Professor (IUCSAL)
Director, Fascia Research Group
Division of Neurophysiology, Ulm University
Ulm, Germany.

Reviewers

Bethany M. Ward, M.B.A., L.M.B.T.
Certified Advanced Rolfer™, Rolf Movement® Practitioner
Faculty, Rolf Institute® of Structural Integration
Advisor and Past President, Ida P. Rolf Research Foundation
Director, ActionPotential, Inc.
Durham, North Carolina, United States.

Ruth Werner, B.C.T.M.B.
Continuing Education Provider, Author
Director, Werner Workshops
Waldport, Oregon, United States.

Online Resources

Scan the code or visit http://advanced-trainings.com/amt1/ for supplementary online resources, including:

- Online video library
- Professional Continuing Education and CMA credit options
- Teacher and student classroom resources
- Free myofascial webinars
- Forum and social media links for questions and dialog about Advanced Myofascial Techniques
- Offers and discounts from Primal Pictures, Advanced-Trainings.com, and others mentioned in this book.

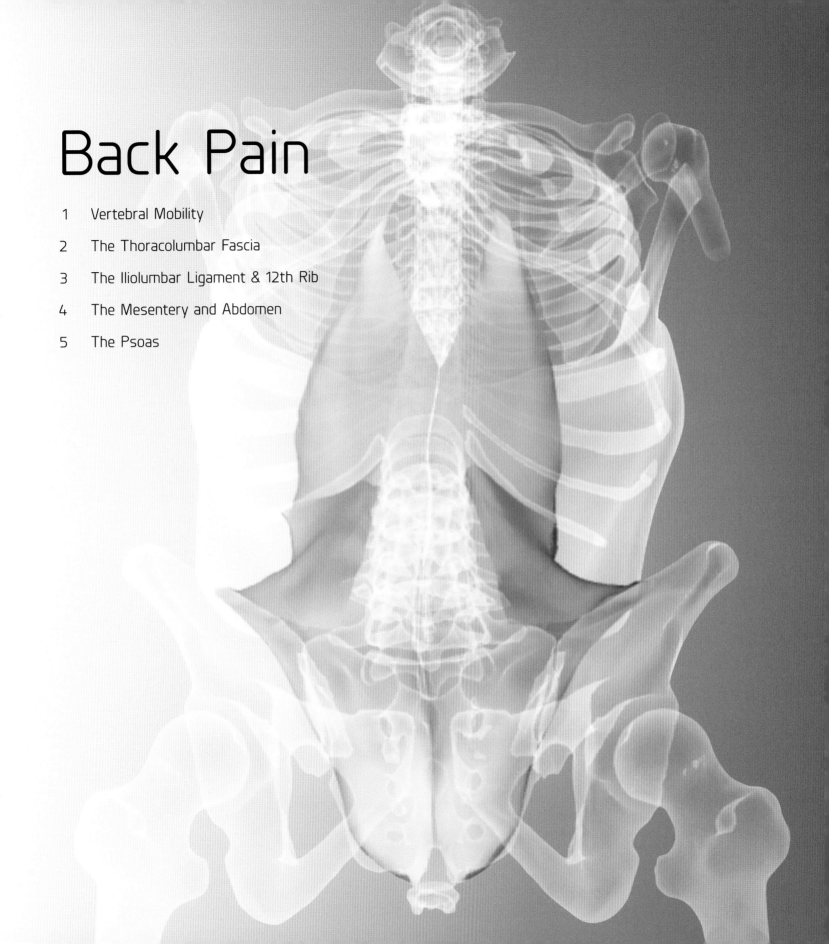

Back Pain

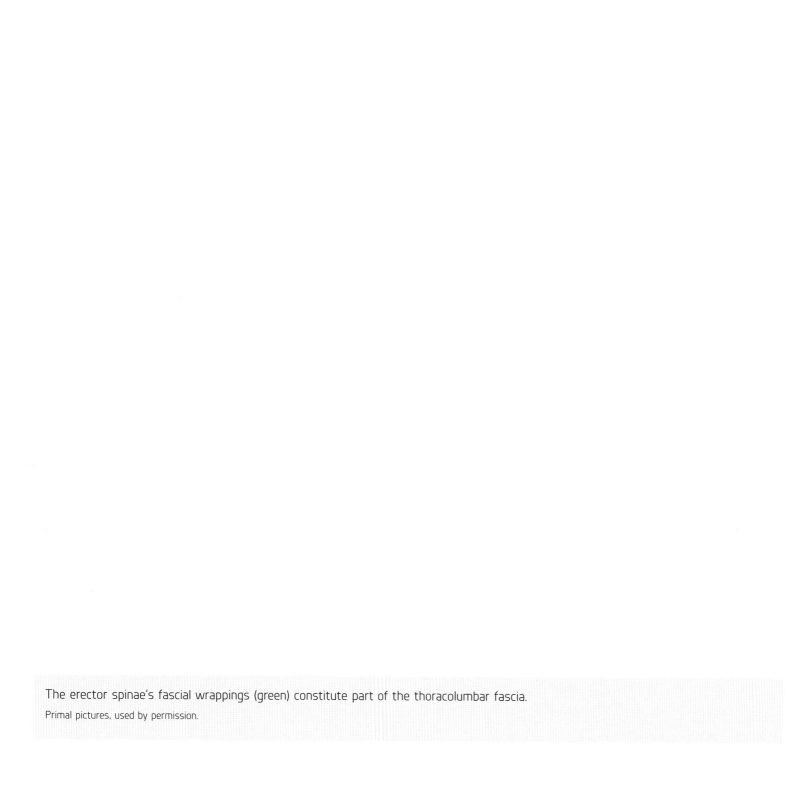

The erector spinae's fascial wrappings (green) constitute part of the thoracolumbar fascia.

Vertebral Mobility

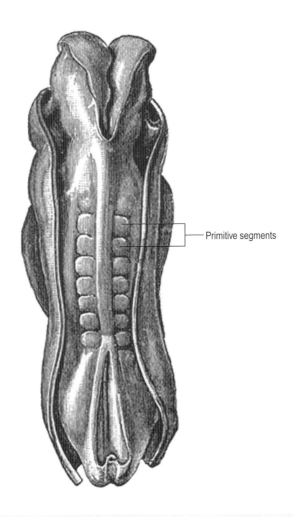

Figure 1.1

The somites (or segments) of the emerging spine in an embryo at about 20 days of development; 1/12" (2.11mm) in length. Not only do somites become the individual vertebrae, but they also give rise to much of the musculoskeletal and connective tissues at their corresponding level of the body.

Primitive segments

There is nothing in the body that quite compares to the spine. Its centrality, size, and crucial role in support and movement, as well as its integral relationship with the central and peripheral nervous systems all mean that when we work with the spine, we have our hands on one of the most important structures in our work.

The importance of the spine is reflected in the way we use its name in everyday speech. Roget's lists the word *spine* as a synonym for "core," "foundation," "basis" (as in the spine of his philosophy), as well as for "perseverance," "decisiveness," "nerve," and "fearlessness" (1). Think about what it means to "have a backbone," or to be "spineless"; linguistically, we relate our spine to our very character, strength, and human resilience.

Embryologically and evolutionarily, the spine's precursor (the notochord) is one of the first structures to distinguish itself from the matrix of rapidly dividing cells in a developing vertebrate (Figure 1.1). After just 20 days, a human embryo has segmented its midline into the somites that will become our individual vertebrae. These proto-vertebrae give rise to other structures as well: many of our musculoskeletal and connective tissue structures develop outward from this longitudinal arrangement of cells as we grow, making the spine the root structure for much of our musculoskeletal form (2).

The spine and vertebrae are directly involved in several of the most common client complaints, including:

- Rib pain (since the ribs articulate directly with the vertebrae at the ligamentous costovertebral joints).
- Neck pain or injury, including whiplash (the neck being the uppermost section of the spine, and thus dependent on the supporting sections below for its stability and ease).

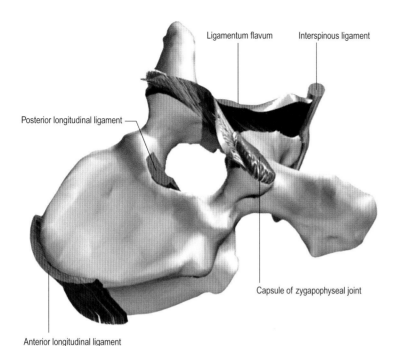

Ligamentum flavum Interspinous ligament

Posterior longitudinal ligament

Capsule of zygapophyseal joint

Anterior longitudinal ligament

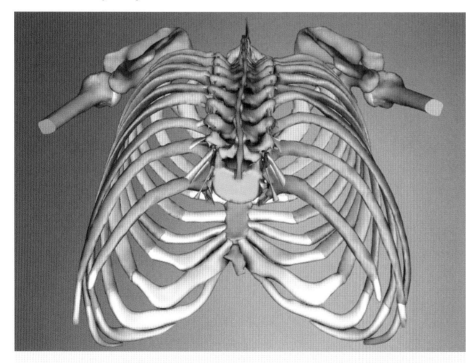

Figures 1.2/1.3

Normal vertebral mobility can be diminished by inelastic or undifferentiated soft tissues around the spine and ribs. In addition to the spinal ligaments and joint capsules shown in Figure 1.2, muscles and myofascial structures of the spine (such as the thoracolumbar fascia, the multifidi, erectors, etc.) can also affect vertebral mobility.

- Sacroiliac issues (the sacrum and its paired sacroiliac joints being the base of support for the entire spine, and in turn subject to the forces of flexing, extending, bending, and twisting coming from the long lever of the spine above).
- Sciatic pain (especially axial sciatic pain, as discussed in "Sciatic Pain," *Advanced Myofascial Techniques, Volume 1*, p 107).
- And of course, back pain itself (which affects nine in ten people at some point in their lives (3)), as well as other spine-related issues such as scoliosis, spondylolisthesis, etc.

The mobility of the spine, both of individual vertebra and of the entire structure, plays a role in each of these issues. Since "increased options for movement" is one of the primary goals of our Advanced Myofascial Techniques work (4), we can often play a helpful role for our clients with these spine-related issues.

Vertebral motion disparities

Coupled-motion biomechanics is a set of principles that have influenced numerous manual therapy disciplines (5), including osteopathic manipulation, physical therapy, Rolfing, structural integration, rehabilitative massage, and other manual therapy modalities.

At the risk of oversimplification, I'll attempt a brief overview. The spine's overall mobility is determined by the combined smaller motions between individual vertebrae. This motion between vertebrae can be restricted by their surrounding ligaments and myofascia (Figure 1.2), and in the thoracic spine, by soft tissues surrounding the costovertebral joints (Figure 1.3). When these soft tissues are elastic and differentiated enough to allow unrestricted vertebral motion, normal activities like breathing, walking, and bending will cause the vertebrae to move in all three dimensions in relationship to their neighbors.

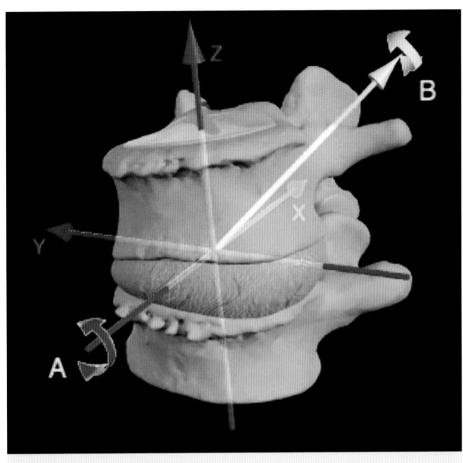

Figure 1.4

One model of lumbar vertebral motion, illustrating the coupled relationship of sidebending (A) with rotation around an oblique axis (B). While it is generally accepted that motion of a vertebra in one dimension is coupled with motion in all dimensions, there is a lack of agreement between different theoretical models (and between different 3D studies) about the normal direction of coupling.

Most biomechanics authors (though not all) agree that due to their bony shapes and complex soft-tissue interconnections, these movements are often coupled, so that movement in one plane is automatically accompanied by motions in the other two planes (Figure 1.4) (6). According to one moderately large study (*n* = 369) physiotherapists of diverse backgrounds view coupling biomechanics as an important part of their hands-on approach, with more than 85 percent of therapists surveyed indicating that lumbar coupling biomechanics were "very important" or "important" in their application of manual therapy (7).

Interestingly, in spite of the importance placed on biomechanical coupling by many practitioners, there is little agreement about the optimal direction of this coupling, with several conflicting models of "normal" spinal biomechanics in existence. For example, some models (such as Fryette's Laws) assert that in a neutrally positioned spine, when the lumbars sidebend to the left, they rotate right; others (Lovett) say the opposite (left sidebending is coupled by left rotation); while still others (Roland) say there is no coupled motion in this situation at all (8). Real-world studies of asymptomatic 3D spinal motion have not settled these disputes, as different studies have shown "variable" and contradictory results, particularly at different levels of the spine (9). One likely possibility (which has been documented in coupled motion controversies about other parts of the body (10) is that healthy individuals' joints do not all seem to move in the same ways, probably due to differences in bone and joint shape. One recent overview of biomechanical theory concludes that although cervical dynamics are similar from person to person, "no consistent coupling behavior has been demonstrated in the thoracic or lumbar spine" (11). In other words, in spite of being an important aspect of many hands-on modalities, some of

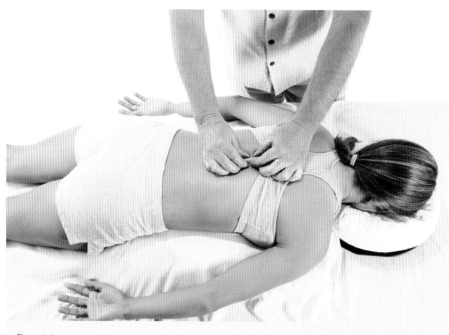

Figure 1.5

Assessing the rotational freedom of a group of vertebrae in the Vertebral Mobility Technique.

the fundamental "laws" of spinal biomechanics don't seem to apply in many cases.

As practitioners, where does this contradiction and uncertainty leave us? Speaking only for myself, after having studied, used, and taught Greenman-influenced (12) coupled-motion biomechanics for many years, my approach has become more pragmatic than theoretical. My current working hypothesis is that mobility is indeed vitally important for pain-free, easy functioning but that concepts of "normal" or "correct" biomechanical motion are probably less predictably meaningful. As a guiding principle, this idea might be restated *simply as when things don't move enough, and in different directions, they don't feel good*; when we can help them move again, they feel better.

Vertebral Mobility Technique

A good example of this simple principle at work is the Vertebral Mobility Technique. Because it allows the practitioner to feel, see, and address vertebral mobility restrictions, and because it can quiet and focus the client's attention, we use this technique in our Advanced Myofascial Techniques trainings before performing other work with the spine or ribcage. On its own or in combination with other techniques, it is indicated as assessment and preparation for many of the spine-related conditions listed at the beginning of this article.

Standing beside your prone client, gently but firmly grasp the spinous processes of several thoracic vertebrae (Figure 1.5). When the spinal erectors are very large, the spinous processes can be deep and hard to grasp; if this is the case, use a deeper touch, or the sides of your fingers, rather than fingertips alone.

Use the spinous process as a handle to gently move the group of vertebrae from side to side, using small, rhythmic motions to rock this group of vertebrae within their attachments to

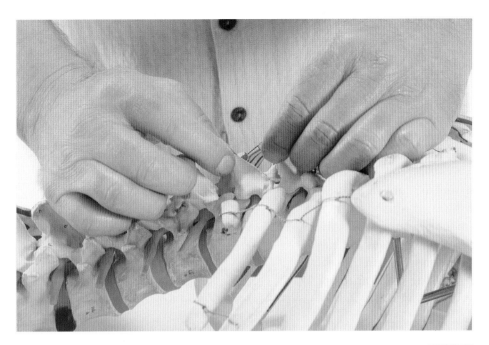

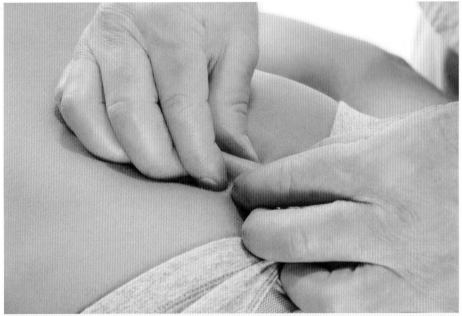

Figures 1.6/1.7
Assessing and mobilizing a pair of vertebrae in the Vertebral Mobility Technique.

the surrounding ribs (Figure 1.3). Begin delicately, feeling for the amount of subtle mobility possible with very little force. Is the motion and resistance the same left and right? Don't confuse any apparent misalignment of the spinous process with their mobility—a vertebra's spinous process can be crooked or bent to the side, largely independent of its mobility. Does movement vary from place to place? Investigate this subtle rotational movement throughout the spine, noting restrictions as you find them. Often, these small, focused movements will result in more vertebral movement, probably as a result of mechanoreceptor stimulation, postural reflex shift, and increased proprioception.

After assessing subtle mobility, you can begin to move a bit more vigorously, still within you client's level of comfort, of course. Use a fuller, firmer rocking motion on any areas where you find restrictions. Use caution if any of the usual contraindications to deep work apply—in particular, suspected osteoporosis (see Chapter 7, *The Ribs*), recent injuries, or acute disc issues. But in most cases, the motion can be spirited, strong, and adventurous throughout the lumbar and thoracic spine. The vertebrae are firmly held by their ligamentous and articular connections, so you can use the body's momentum to assess and increase their side-to-side mobility.

Feel both for grouped restrictions and, by moving single vertebrae against each other, for pairs of vertebrae that are fixed together (Figures 1.6 and 1.7). Go back and forth between these global and local levels, feeling also for whole-spine harmonics (waves that move all the way up and down), and for the small-scale jiggling of individually immobile vertebrae.

With care, you can also apply this technique to many of the cervical vertebrae, gently feeling for side-to-side mobility of each neck vertebra that you can palpate. A face cradle or tabletop bolstering system is necessary, so that the neck is not rotated to one side.

This technique assesses and improves the rotational freedom of the vertebrae.[1] This doesn't imply that the other directions of movement aren't important; we use different techniques to assess and mobilize those motions as well. Especially with issues such as scoliosis, or long-term fixations, you're likely to identify areas with this assessment that you'll want to address with other techniques. But even by itself, this assessment and preparatory technique can be quite effective and satisfying. As a client, the experience of having each of your vertebrae mobilized in this way can be deeply relaxing, leaving you primed and ready for the rest of your session.

Key points: Vertebral Mobility Technique

Indications include:

- Back pain or mobility restrictions.
- Spine-related issues such as pain or mobility restrictions in the neck, ribs, sacroiliac joints, etc.
- Whiplash and other injuries.
- Axial sciatic pain, etc.

Purpose

- Assess mobility restrictions to inform later techniques.
- Quiet and focus the client's attention in preparation for other work.
- Increase vertebral proprioception and options for rotational movement.

Instructions

1. Gently but firmly grip the spinous processes of the vertebrae.
2. Beginning with subtle movement, assess side-to-side movement (vertebral rotation).
3. Assess and mobilize both local and global mobility.
4. Optionally, use larger, fuller movements for any persistent restriction.

References

[1] Roget's *21st Century Thesaurus, 3rd edition*. (2009). Philip Lief Group.

[2] Sadler, T.W. (2012) *Langman's Medical Embryology*. 12th ed. Lippincott Williams & Wilkins. p. 63.

[3] Frymoyer, J.D. (1988) Back pain and sciatica. *New England Journal of Medicine*. 318. p. 291–300.

[4] Luchau, T. (2015) *Advanced Myofascial Techniques, vol. 1*. Handspring Publishing. p. 8.

[5] Cook, C. and Showalter, B. (2004) A survey on the importance of lumbar coupling biomechanics in physiotherapy practice. *Manual Therapy*. 9. p. 164–172.

[6] DeStephano, L. (2010) Greenman's *Principles of Manual Medicine*. 4th ed. Lippincott Williams & Wilkins.

[7] Cook & Showalter (2004) ibid, 167.

[8] Cook & Showalter (2004) ibid, 165.

[9] Cook & Showalter (2004) ibid, 166.

[10] Bozkurt, M. et al. (2008) Axial rotation and mediolateral translation of the fibula during passive plantar flexion. *Foot Ankle Int*. 29(5). p. 502–507

[11] Parsons, J. and Marcer, N. (2006) *Osteopathy: Models for Diagnosis, Treatment and Practice*. Elsevier Health Sciences. p. 36.

[12] DeStephano, L. (2010) ibid.

[13] Novella, S. (2009) *Chiropractic: A Brief Overview, Part I*. http://www.sciencebasedmedicine.org/chiropractic-a-brief-overview-part-i/. [Accessed December 2015]

[14] Kaptchuk, T.J. and Eisenberg, D.M. (1998) Chiropractic: Origins, controversies, and contributions. *Archives of Internal Medicine*. 158(20). p. 2215–2224. doi:10.1001/archinte.158.20.2215.

[15] Clinical and Professional Chiropractic Education: A Position Statement. *The European-South African Education Collaboration*. http://www.ifec.net/wp-content/uploads/2015/05/Educational-Statements-june-2015.pdf. [Accessed December 2015]

Picture credits

Figure 1.1 Artist: Henry Vandyke Carter, from *Henry Gray's Anatomy of the Human Body* (1918). Image is in the public domain.

Figures 1.2, 1.3, and 1.4 Primal Pictures, used by permission.

Figures 1.5, 1.6, and 1.7 Advanced-Trainings.com.

---

1 For the sake of clarity, when we work with vertebrae in this way, we are affecting the soft-tissue restrictions that limit mobility. We are not performing osseous adjustments, or treating vertebral rotations or subluxations in the way a chiropractor might.

Study Guide

Vertebral Mobility

1 **What vertebral motion is being assessed in the Vertebral Mobility Technique?**

a flexion
b extension
c sidebending
d rotation

2 **According to the text, how does a misaligned spinous process affect mobility in the Vertebral Mobility Technique?**

a vertebral motion is usually greater in the same direction as process misalignment
b vertebral motion is usually greater in the opposite direction of process misalignment
c vertebral motion is greater on same side as process according to Lovett, opposite according to Fryette
d vertebral motion is largely independent of process alignment

3 **How does the author suggest beginning the Vertebral Mobility Technique?**

a with very little force
b in the lumbar spine
c in the neck
d with large movements

4 **The text states that the spine's overall mobility is determined by:**

a sidebending freedom between individual vertebrae
b the combined motions between individual vertebrae
c rotational freedom between individual vertebrae
d the alignment of the spinous processes

5 **Which of these is most congruent with the author's working hypothesis on coupled vertebral motion?**

a When vertebrae don't sidebend enough in the same direction as rotation, they don't feel good
b When vertebrae don't sidebend enough in the opposite direction as rotation, they don't feel good
c When vertebrae sidebend they shouldn't rotate; if they do, they don't feel good
d When vertebrae don't move enough, and in different directions, they don't feel good

For Answer Keys, visit www.Advanced-Trainings.com/v2key/

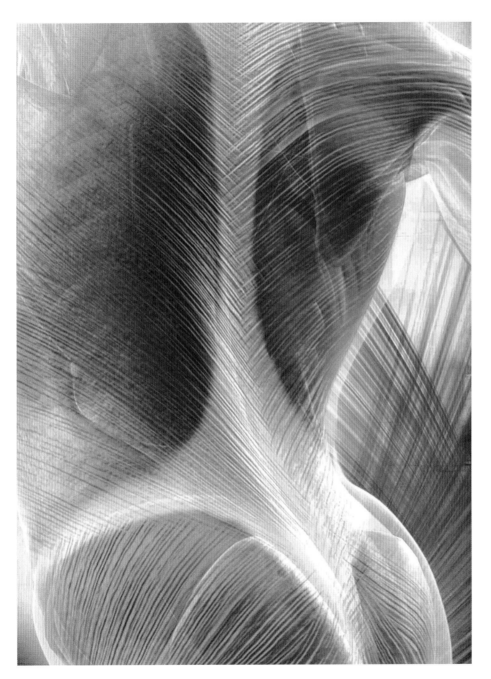

To be human is to have back pain. Back pain is one of the most common physical disorders that humans endure. It affects about 90 percent of people at some point in their lives (1), and ranks as the leading cause of disability worldwide (2).

Low back pain (LBP) has been with us for as long as we have had backs, and for just as long, humans have been seeking to understand and relieve back pain. The oldest known writings on surgery—the 3500-year-old Edwin Smith Papyrus from Ancient Egypt—include tests and treatments for back sprain. In more recent medical history, different mechanisms have been thought to be the primary source of back pain at different times. The changing theories about LBP's primary cause have included referred sacroiliac joint pain (3) and nerve inflammation (a popular explanation in the early 1900s); "muscular rheumatism" (fibromyalgia) (4) and psychological issues such as "hysteria" (5) (1920s–1930s); quadratus lumborum (QL) spasm (until the 1950s); disc issues (1930s–1990s; discussed in more detail later in this chapter); transversus abdominis strength (1990s) (6); multifidus size (2000s) (7); and the more recent emphasis on "core stability" (in the last decade).

While many of these theories have proven to be important pieces of the back pain puzzle, up to 85 percent of back pain cases still have no known cause (8), and the search for understanding and effective treatment continues. Recently, a number of researchers have identified another contributor to many kinds of previously unexplained LBP: the highly innervated thoracolumbar fascia (TLF); we'll discuss the specifics below.

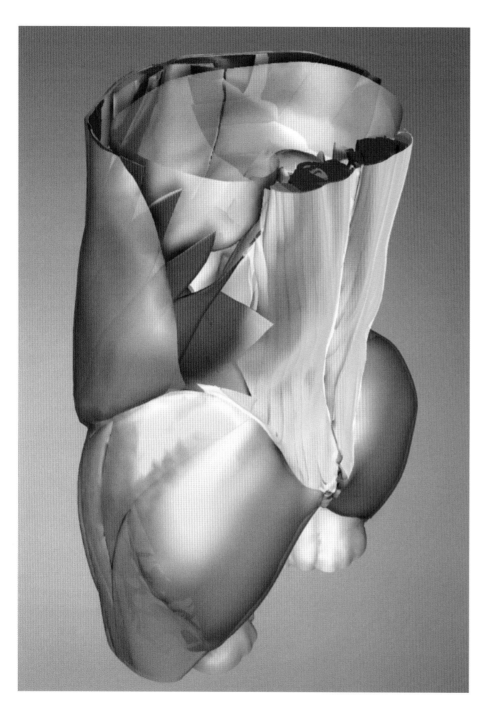

The thoracolumbar fascia's role in LBP

The sensitive TLF (also known as the *lumbodorsal fascia*) covers and separates many of the muscle groupings that lie posterior to the spine. From behind, anatomy texts often depict it as a diamond-shaped connective tissue structure lying over the lower back, connecting the gluteal fascia to the latissimus dorsi (Figure 2.1). However, from other angles, it becomes clear that this structure is much more complex. Multiple layers wrap three-dimensionally around the various structures of the low back (Figures 2.2 and 2.3), and extend from the base of the neck (where it is contiguous with the deep cervical fascia) to the sacrum and iliac crests of the pelvis. Its different layers adhere to the processes of the lumbar vertebrae and spinal ligaments along the midline of the back, and it adheres to the ribs laterally. The TLF wraps around and connects several of the structures thought to be responsible for LBP, such as the spinal ligaments, the QL, and the transversospinalis muscles (including the erectors and multifidi). It also interconnects other key muscles involved in back pain such as the transverse abdominis, the obliques and, via its upper end, the diaphragm.

The recent increase in the awareness of fascia's role in sensation and pain perception has stimulated research showing that pain-signaling free nerve endings and mechanoreceptors in the back's TLF are more abundant than previously thought, and that the TLF is significantly thicker in those with LBP than in those without (9). Other research has shown that there is less gliding between the deeper layers of the TLF in people with LBP (10). This suggests that our method's goals of increased fascial elasticity and layer differentiation (see Volume I: Chapter 2, *Understanding Fascial Change*) may be part of why manual therapy has been observed to help

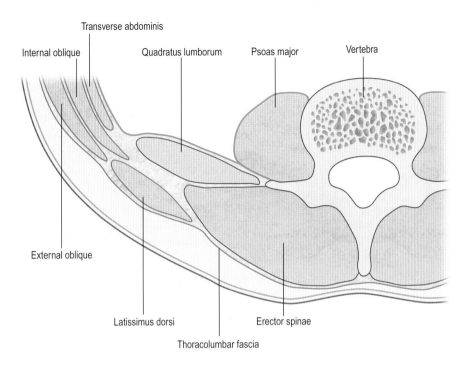

Transverse abdominis

Internal oblique   Quadratus lumborum   Psoas major   Vertebra

External oblique

Latissimus dorsi   Erector spinae

Thoracolumbar fascia

Figures 2.1/2.2/2.3

The multi-layered thoracolumbar fascia (TLF, also known as the lumbodorsal fascia), shown in green in Figures 2.2 and 2.3. A tough, fibrous, and multilayered confluence of fascial sheets connecting the lower limbs to their upper limb counterparts on the opposite side, it is highly innervated and plays a role in many cases of back pain. The TLF wraps and connects many of the low back structures involved in low back pain, including those labeled here, and attaches to the psoas major fascia as well as the spinous and transverse processes of the vertebrae.

LBP, both anecdotally in the practice room, and statistically in back-pain research (11).

Because the sensitive yet strong TLF diagonally joins each leg to its opposite-side arm, it is an important structure in the mechanical and proprioceptive control of walking, running, throwing, and all contralateral motions. As a whole-body connector, it can be directly involved in many client conditions, including:

- Low- and mid-back pain
- Recurring tightness in the thoracic spine or low back
- Spinal stiffness and restricted rotation or flexion
- Inhibited contralateral arm/leg motion, and
- Limited rib or back motion in diaphragmatic breathing.

The TLF is also indirectly implicated in many other conditions, including hip or sacroiliac pain (12), as well as in suboccipital headaches or plantar fasciitis, via its indirect fascial connections to those regions (13).

Iliac Crest Technique

We will prepare for our work with the low back's fascia by starting with the iliac crests. It is along these thin, bony ridges that the layers of the TLF find their inferolateral attachments to bone; so when we work these attachments, we are also working the conjoined fascial attachments of the transverse abdominis, the internal and external obliques, as well as the iliocostalis, the largest and most lateral of the spinal erectors. The iliac crests are the stop-over place for these and many other soft tissue connections, from both above and below. Since our focus is on preparing for low back work, we will emphasize the superior aspect of these bony ridges where the low back structures attach.

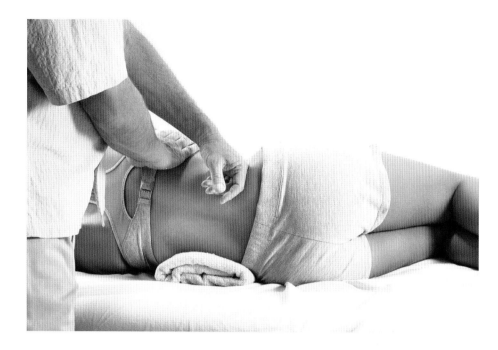

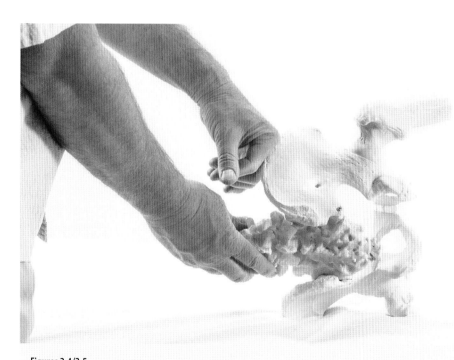

Figures 2.4/2.5

The Iliac Crest Technique. Gently use the knuckles of a soft fist to work the attachments of the TLF and other structures along the length of the iliac crests. Glide slowly to prepare the outer layers; use static pressure on deeper layers.

Using a soft fist, feel for the bony ridge of the iliac crest. Use the furrow between two of your knuckles as a way to wrap around the crest's ridge slightly (Figures 2.4 and 2.5). On many clients with long-term low back pain or strain, you will find thick, dense fascial buildup here. Starting at the lateral-most part of the hip crest, sink in slowly, feeling for the tissue to soften in response. By waiting for this response, we are evoking a reduction in the resting tone of the fascia's associated muscles via a Golgi tendon organ reflex (14). This allows our work to have a much greater effect, as by waiting, we affect much more than the small area we are contacting with our soft fist. This reduction in tone is therapeutic in and of itself; it also serves to prepare the body for the more direct work with the lumbar sections of the TLF (which will be addressed in the next technique).

Once you have felt the tissue here soften slightly in response to your static, patient pressure, you can begin to slowly glide along the crest to a new area. Wait here for a tissue response; its softening will allow you to glide to the next area. As you glide medially along the crest, you will encounter the more muscular attachments of the QL and the iliocostalis. Slow down even more. Perhaps take a more superficial layer, at least for your first pass. Continue this process of waiting for a response in each place, until you have reached the posterior superior iliac spine—the posterior terminus of the iliac crest. Repeat at a slightly deeper level; or, move on to the next technique.

Key points: Iliac Crest Technique

Indications include:

- Low- and mid-back pain.
- Recurring tightness in the thoracic spine or low back.
- Spinal stiffness and restricted rotation or flexion.
- Inhibited contralateral arm/leg motion.
- Limited rib or back motion in diaphragmatic breathing.

Purpose

- Increase layer differentiation and elasticity of the TLF.
- Reduce resting tone of the muscles attaching to the iliac crests
- Prepare tissues for deeper low back work.

Instructions

With the client in a side lying position:

- Use the knuckles of a soft fist to feel for the superficial layers of the TLF on the superior aspect of the iliac crests. Wait with static pressure for the tissues to soften.
- Use this softening to slowly glide lateral to medial, until reaching the PSIS.
- Repeat with progressively deeper layers, eventually feeling for the TFL attachments on the iliac crests themselves.

Thoracolumbar Fascia Technique

Your work along the iliac crests addressed the inferior attachments of the TLF, which will make your work with the rest of the low back easier and more effective. The TLF is composed of dense, fibrous connective tissue layers that are separated by thin layers of loose connective tissue; these thin layers normally allow the dense layers to glide against one another during trunk and limb motion. As mentioned, less gliding between the layers here has been correlated with lower back pain (15). We will address each layer of the TLF in turn, restoring differentiation and elasticity as we go.

Superficial and Posterior Layers

There are several outer layers in the low back—the skin, the various layers of superficial fascia, and several layers of deeper fascia underneath. These include the posterior (outermost) layer of the TLF, which covers the erector/multifidus group, and gives rise to the latissimus dorsi that connects the back to the arm (Figures 2.1 and 2.3).

Using a soft fist, sink into the space between the iliac crest and the 12th rib. Use a light enough touch that you can easily glide from the lateral to medial aspects of this space, using your slow, patient friction to move each layer in turn. Do not use lubricant. The friction itself is the therapeutic tool that increases layer differentiation. Make sure your pressure is comfortable for the client; the TLF sub-layers here are all richly innervated, and are sometimes even more sensitive than the deeper layers underneath. Feel for an increase in tissue elasticity and easier gliding of one layer upon another. Repeat this process until you have worked the surface tissues of the entire span between the pelvis and the ribs.

Once you have prepared the outer layers with several lighter passes, you can engage your client's active movement. Ask for slow, active motions from the participant—for example, "Let your knee slowly come towards your chest," or "Very slowly, reach up above your head." Make sure your client is breathing easily. Engaging the limbs and breath in this way will broaden the effects of your work, and evoke more powerful Golgi and nervous system responses.

See video of the Thoracolumbar Fascia Technique at www.a-t.tv/sb06

Erector and Multifidus Layer

The spinal erectors and multifidi lie between the TLF's posterior and middle layers. Many practitioners are accustomed to addressing the erectors from their posterior aspect in a prone client, which is how these large, thick muscles are depicted in most anatomy illustrations. However, with your client in a side-lying position, gravity enables a different approach. Begin with a soft fist to feel for the lateral edge of this large group of muscles (Figure 2.6).

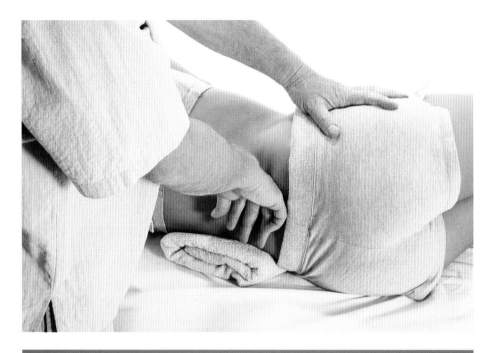

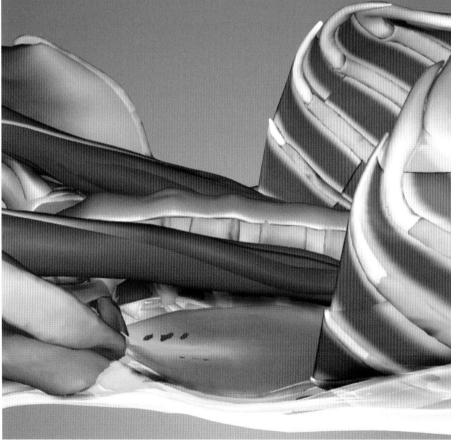

The entire muscle group will be several inches thick, and it constitutes the bulk of the muscle mass next to the lumbar spine (Figures 2.7 and 2.9). Rather than sliding on the surface, as we did with the previous fascial layers, sink in to the thick lateral aspect of the erector group (Figure 2.7). You will need to be positioned above your client in order to use gravity, so your table will be quite low, or you may need to kneel on your table.

If there is enough space between your client's ribs and pelvis, instead of using a soft fist, you can carefully use your forearm to work the erectors' lateral aspects (Figure 2.8). Be extremely gentle and cautious with the forearm—avoid using the point of your elbow; instead, use the broad, flat surface of your ulna. Avoid any pain—if your client is not comfortable with your pressure or pace, more preparation and a slower approach are indicated. Use your forearm to feel, more than to manipulate.

Wait for a softening of this thick muscular layer. Your touch is static, deep, and perceptive. You do not need to glide or move to affect the TLF here—your static pressure is quite effective at evoking sensation and change, both within the muscles and in their enveloping fasciae.

As a variation, you can ask your client for slow active client movement, as you did with the outer layers. This will move the fascia under your static touch and help with neuromuscular re-education as you coach your client to find new, more refined ways to initiate movement. At this deeper level, the movements must be very slow and deliberate since they will intensify your client's sensations. Be extra sensitive. Cue your client to make minute movements, as you work very slowly. Motions might include slow hip flexion or extension; reaching with arms; or pelvic tucking and rocking. If you are patient and sensitive, you can work very

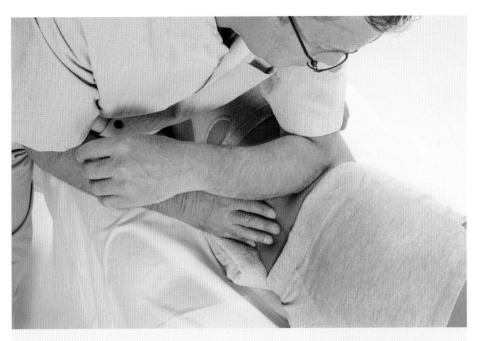

Figures 2.6/2.7/2.8

The Thoracolumbar Fascia Technique works three-dimensionally to differentiate the various layers of the TLF, from superficial to deep, as to wraps around the thick muscle mass of the erectors (Figure 2.7). Figure 2.8 shows very gentle work with the ulna on the erector layers. Use caution around the sharp and sensitive transverse processes of the spine, as well as the ends of the floating ribs.

deeply here, as your client's slow, deliberate movements both free fascial layers and increase proprioception of the limbs' connection to the spine.

Quadratus Lumborum Layer

Just anterior to the erectors, or deeper into the body, you will find the QL between the middle and anterior layers of the TLF (Figures 2.3 and 2.9). The QL is a key stabilizer of the trunk/pelvis relationship; as a postural muscle, it is active in bending, balancing, walking, and breathing. Well known to manual therapy practitioners as a crucial structure to include when addressing back pain, the QL and the fascia around it (on average, the fascia around a muscle has about six times more nerve endings than muscle tissue itself) (16) can be a source of many kinds of back discomfort.

To find the QL and its fascia, use the Iliac Crest Technique to follow the crest medially until you encounter the attachments of the QL. From here, you can begin to use your two thumbs together (Figure 2.10) to isolate the QL layer. Do not hyperextend your thumbs or apply excessive pressure with them. Use static pressure and active client movements, as you did with the other layers. Work the QL from its attachments in the iliac crest to its insertion on the 12th rib. Breathing and hip motions will be particularly relevant.

Key points: Thoracolumbar Fascia Technique

Indications include:
- Low- and mid-back pain.
- Recurring tightness in the thoracic spine or low back.
- Spinal stiffness and restricted rotation or flexion.
- Inhibited contralateral arm/leg motion.
- Limited rib or back motion in diaphragmatic breathing.

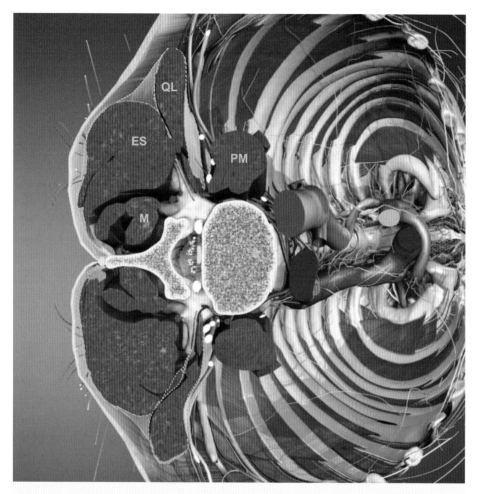

Figure 2.9

The deepest layers of the TLF (green) wrap the quadratus lumborum (QL), which is anterior or deep to the erector spinae (ES). The multifidi (M) and psoas major (PM) are also shown.

Purpose
- Differentiate and increase glide between the many layers of the TLF.
- Increase options for movement in the spine and torso.
- Refine the initiation of limb movement, and increase the proprioceptive awareness of limb motion's connection to the spine.

Instructions
With the client in a side lying position:
1. Use a soft fist to sink into the space between the 12th rib and iliac crest.
2. With static touch (not gliding), wait for a change in tissue elasticity and muscle tonus, then cue active motions.
3. Alternatively, gently use your forearm for deeper layers.

Movements
With special attention to the gradual initiation of movement, ask for slow, active:
- hip flexion (knee to chest), hip abduction/adduction.
- shoulder flexion/abduction.
- pelvic tilt.
- breathing.

Considerations and Precautions
- Avoid medial pressure onto the transverse processes and the ends of the floating ribs.
- Use caution and a very gradual approach with disc issues to avoid destabilization.
- Strong LBP of sudden or frequent onset is probably cause for referral to a specialist for evaluation.

Considerations

When properly applied, the work described here has proven to be very safe and effective. It has been taught to thousands of practitioners on several continents over the last two decades in our continuing education trainings. However, some important considerations apply:

- In the side-lying work, be mindful of the ends of the floating ribs and the transverse processes of the vertebrae, both of which are

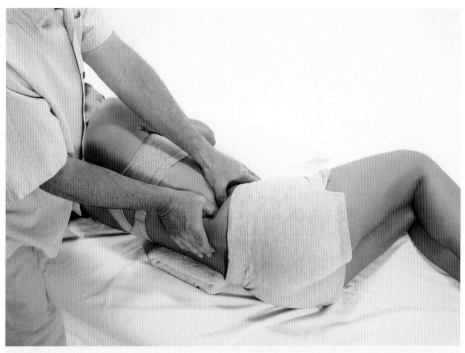

Figure 2.10

Careful use of the thumbs is one option when working with the deep quadratus lumborum layer. Keep your two thumbs together, avoid hyperextending any joints, and check with your client about comfort. Adding breath and slow hip movement can increase effectiveness of this and the other TLF techniques.

sensitive, and could be injured by incautious work. Avoid putting pressure directly on the transverse processes—there are stories of overly aggressive lumbar work bruising the tissue here by pushing it against the pointed processes. Stay in touch with your client's comfort level; do not try to "rub away" any bumps or apparent knots that you might find—they might be bone.

- These techniques are most effective on mild to moderate chronic back pain. Recent back injuries or surgery are usually contraindications to the direct approach described here, at least until the tissues have healed (although with care, experienced practitioners can often adapt these ideas for recent back injuries. One key is to apply the techniques gently and gradually, noting responses between sessions). Older, healed injuries and surgeries often respond very favorably to these techniques.

- Strong LBP of sudden or frequent onset is probably cause for referral to rehabilitation or complementary specialists, such as a physical therapist, chiropractor, or physician, since LBP may need more care than most manual therapists can typically provide, as LBP can sometimes signal serious medical issues.

- Disc issues: until recently, intervertebral disc issues (bulging, herniation, degeneration, and so on) were the favored explanation for many types of LBP, with discectomy surgery increasing in popularity tremendously after its introduction in the 1930s (leading some authors to refer to the decades that followed as the "dynasty of the disc" (17)). However, since the 1980s, there has been less emphasis on disc issues as a major cause of LBP, as more recent research has shown that most disc issues are a relatively uncommon cause of pain. Most disc issues are asymptomatic, and while more than 60 percent of people over age 40 show evidence of disc degeneration, a much lower percentage have any related pain (18). Nevertheless, I do not recommend using these techniques with disc issues until you are very familiar with their application and can reliably gauge the appropriate pressure, duration, and response. The danger in working with disc issue patients is that releasing their compensatory muscular and fascial tension too quickly, or in an unbalanced way, could aggravate or further destabilize a fragile pattern. Play it safe and refer these clients to a specialist, or work under a specialist's close supervision until you have gained enough experience to competently address the trickier situation of disc issues and unstable LBP.

Summary

At the beginning of this chapter, we listed some of the many mechanisms that have been thought to be responsible for back pain through the ages. While all of these factors may contribute to LBP, and treatments based on them may all give relief in individual cases, none of these theories have proven to be a silver bullet cure-all, nor has any one approach been consistently effective with a majority of LBP suffers. In a survey of the leading back pain theories published over the last 100 years, the authors conclude that "today we know that for the majority of low back pain cases, a specific etiology [cause] cannot be determined" (19).

In spite of this, many back pain sufferers do find relief in hands-on work (as well as other approaches). Our increased understanding of the TLF's sensitivity and role in back pain is a significant addition to our knowledge base, and this gives manual therapists new tools to help many clients' back pain that has not responded to other treatments. Like most of the LBP theories discussed earlier, the ideas discussed in this chapter add a piece to our overall understanding—even if none of these theories have yet proven that they are sufficiently effective to make back pain completely obsolete.

References

[1] Frymoyer, J.D. (1988) Back pain and sciatica. *New England Journal of Medicine.* 318. p. 291–300.

[2] Institute for Health Metrics and Evaluation (2010) *Global Burden of Disease Study.*

[3] Don Tigney, R. The Sacroiliac Joint. http://www.thelowback.com/history. htm. [Accessed December 2015]

[4] Lutz, G.K. et al. (2003) Looking back on back pain: Trial and error of diagnoses in the 20th Century. *Spine.* 28(16). p. 1899–1905.

[5] Maharty, D.C. (2012) The history of lower back pain: A look back through the centuries. *Primary Care.* 39(3). p. 463–470.

[6] Hodges, P.W. and Richardson, C.A. (1996) Inefficient muscular stabilisation of the lumbar spine associated with low back pain: A motor control evaluation of Transversus Abdominis. *Spine.* 21(22). p. 2640–2650.

[7] Danneels L.A. et al. (2000) CT imaging of trunk muscles in chronic low back pain patients and healthy control subjects. *European Spine Journal.* 9(4). p. 266–272.

[8] Deyo, R. and Weinstein, J. (2001) Low back pain. *New England Journal of Medicine.* 344. p. 363–370.

[9] Langevin H.M. et al. (2009) Ultrasound evidence of altered lumbar connective tissue structure in human subjects with chronic low back pain. *BMC Musculoskeletal Disorders.* 10. p. 151.

[10] Langevin H.M. et al. (2011) Reduced thoracolumbar fascia shear strain in human chronic low back pain. *BMC Musculoskeletal Disorders.* 12. p. 203.

[11] Furlan, A.D. et al. (2008) Massage for low-back pain, *Cochrane Database of Systematic Reviews.* 4 CD001929.

[12] Nickelston, P. (2013) Thoracolumbar fascia: The chronic pain linchpin. *Dynamic Chiropractic.* 31(21). http://www.dynamicchiropractic.com/mpacms/dc/article.php?id=56728. [Accessed December 2015]

[13] Myers, T. (2009) *Anatomy Trains.* Churchill Livingstone.

[14] Schleip, R. (2003) Fascial plasticity: A new neurobiological explanation, Part I. *Journal of Bodywork and Movement Therapies.* 7(1). p. 14.

[15] Langevin, H.M. et al. (2011). ibid. p. 203.

[16] Mitchell, J.H. and Schmidt, R.F. (1977) Cardiovascular reflex control by afferent fibers from skeletal muscle receptors. In: Shepherd, J.T. et al. (eds). *Handbook of Physiology*, Sect. 2, Vol. III, Part 2. Bethesda, MA: American Physiological Society. p. 623–658.

[17] Parisien, R.C. et al. (1998). Ushering in the "dynasty of the disc". *Spine.* 1. 23(21). p. 2363–2366.

[18] MDGuidelines. *Intervertebral Disc Disorders.* Reed Group. (December 2012.)

[19] Lutz, G.K. et al. (August 2003). ibid.

Picture credits

Figure 2.1 Robert Schleip, copyright fascialnet.com, used by permission.
Figures 2.2, 2.7, and 2.9 Primal Pictures, used by permission.
Figures 2.3 based on de Rosa and Porterfield, Advanced-Trainings.com.
Figures 2.4, 2.5, 2.6, 2.8, and 2.10 Advanced-Trainings.com.

Study Guide

The Thoracolumbar Fascia

1 **According to the cited research, how is the thoracolumbar fascia different in those who have low back pain, compared to those who do not?**

a thinner
b tighter
c thicker
d weaker

2 **Along with creating fascial elasticity, what does the chapter list as an additional way that this approach may relieve low back pain?**

a increased layer differentiation
b core strength enhancement
c muscle tone augmentation
d postural re-education

3 **The writing states that the superficial layers of thoracolumbar fascia are often:**

a less sensitive than the deeper layers
b less richly innervated than the muscle tissue they surround
c more sensitive than the deeper layers
d rarely painful

4 **Where does the text suggest working in order to affect the thoracolumbar fascial attachments of the transverse abdominis, the obliques, and the iliocostalis?**

a the lumbar transverse processes
b the thoracic transverse processes
c the lumbar spinous processes
d the iliac crest

5 **How does the text state that the practitioner can evoke a reduction in the resting tone of myofascial tissues?**

a by gliding with lubrication
b by working the spindles in the muscle belly
c by a static touch affecting the Golgi tendon organs
d by working the surrounding ligaments

For Answer Keys, visit www.Advanced-Trainings.com/v2key/

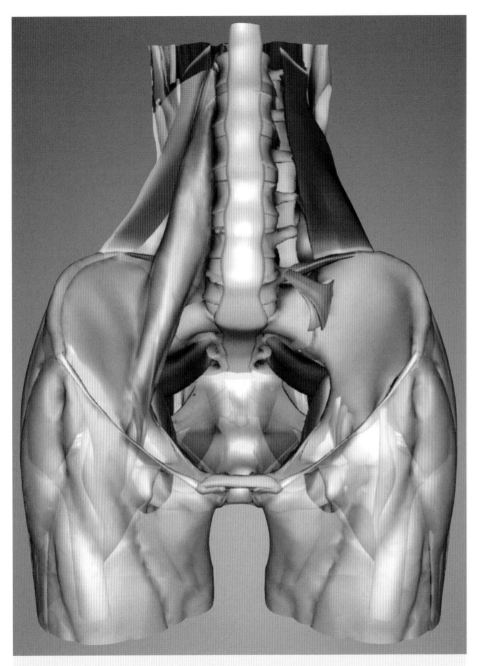

Figure 3.1

The thoracolumbar fascia (or TLF; green) can be a significant a source of low back pain. The iliolumbar ligament (purple) is a thickening in the anterior aspect of this fascia's lower end, where it spans between the lower lumbars and the iliac crest. The iliac fascia is shown surrounding the right iliopsoas; the presacral fascia and fascia lata are also shown (grey).

Deeper isn't necessarily better. But with skill and sensitivity, working deeper can sometimes help in ways that nothing else can. In the previous chapter, *The Thoracolumbar Fascia*, we discussed how strain and micro-tearing in the sensitive thoracolumbar fascia (TLF) has recently been implicated in many kinds of previously unexplained back pain (1). Some of the richly innervated TLF's layers are just below the skin. In our Advanced Myofascial Techniques seminars, we often encourage participants to work with even less pressure, and at an even more superficial layer than many are accustomed to. The powerful results they get with back pain come as a revelation to both practitioners and to their clients.

However, the TLF also has very deep layers and extensions (Figure 3.1), and it makes sense to include these in our work with back pain. In addition to greater sensitivity and skill, deeper work also requires greater tissue preparation and client rapport. The Iliac Crest and the Thoracolumbar Fascia Techniques described in the previous chapter (referenced above) are ideal preparation for the deeper, more specific techniques discussed in this chapter. Use them, or any other approach that helps differentiate tissue layers, relax resting tone, and accustom your client to your touch, before attempting the deeper techniques described here.

More about the thoracolumbar fascia

In the previous chapter, we discussed ways to work with the thoracolumbar fascia (TLF, also known as the lumbodorsal fascia). To recap, the TLF envelops many of the muscular structures of the low back, including the erector spinae and quadratus lumborum (Figure 3.1). It also serves as the connective tissue bridge that connects the abdominal muscles (transversus abdominis, etc.)

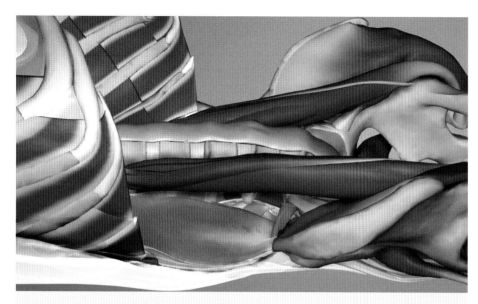

Figure 3.2

The right-side TLF (green) and iliolumbar ligament (purple), shown from the anterolateral direction used in the Iliolumbar Ligament Technique.

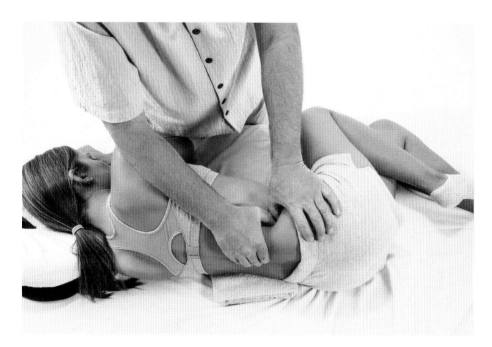

to the spine. Its central position in the body means the TLF connects each arm to its opposite side leg, giving the TLF a crucial force transmission role in contralateral activities such as walking, running, reaching, and throwing.

Working with the TLF is most clearly indicated when clients complain of low- or mid-back stiffness or pain. Back pain has been correlated both to TLF thickness and to lack of sliding between its many layers (2), and hands-on myofascial work has been shown to improve both of these parameters (3).

Deeper TLF work is also useful when the motion of diaphragmatic breathing is posteriorly limited; or when arm/leg cross-patterns (such as a tennis serve, using elliptical trainers, or running or walking) elicit back pain or strain. And because the TLF links upper and lower body as well as left and right, it is indirectly implicated in many other complaints, for example, hip or sacroiliac pain, hamstring pain, abdominal wall issues (such as pain or restriction after cesarean section, hernia repair, etc.), and more.

Iliolumbar Ligament Technique

Back pain linked to the iliolumbar ligaments (ILLs) will often be felt by the client as a deep, dull, generalized ache; or sometimes, as a deep, sharp, sudden pain with spinal sidebending, rotation, or flexion. ILL pain can also refer to the hips, groin, rectum, or genitals (4).

As their name suggests, the iliolumbar ligaments connect the iliac crests to transverse processes of the lowest lumbar vertebrae (Figure 3.2). Rather than being discrete bands of tissue, as they are usually depicted in anatomy illustrations, these ligaments are simply areas of greater thickness and fiber density within the sheet-like TLF. This area's tissue density varies between different individuals, which means our approach for each client will be unique. You'll find these ligaments

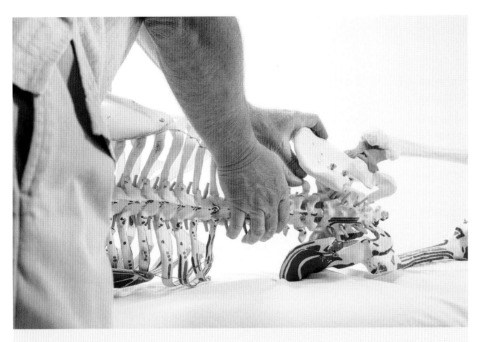

Figures 3.3 (p. 24)/3.4

The anterior approach of the Iliolumbar Ligament Technique. Thoroughly preparing the outer tissue layers of the low back is important before attempting to work at the deep level of the ligaments.

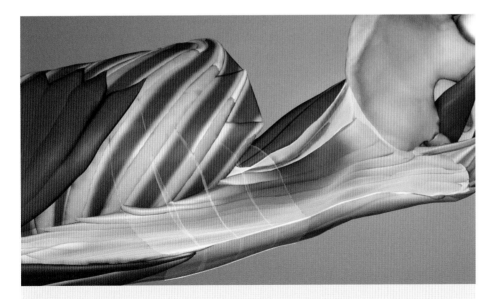

Figure 3.5

The 12th rib (violet) defines the upper margin of the lumbar space. The TLF (green) attaches to this rib, as does the serratus posterior inferior (transparent), the respiratory diaphragm, the quadratus lumborum, and other important structures (not pictured).

are easily accessible on some people, while others may require several sessions of preparatory work—differentiating and increasing the elasticity of each of the outer layers—before you can comfortably access the iliolumbar ligaments.

Some sources even describe the iliolumbar ligaments as too deep to be palpated in living bodies, since they are just inside (slightly anterior to) the iliac crest (Figure 3.2) (5). Although it is probably true that palpating the iliolumbar ligaments is impossible if attempted from a posterior direction (for example, working from behind with a prone client), our thorough preparation of the surrounding tissues and the use of a side-lying position will allow us to gently approach the ligament from an anterolateral direction. This allows us to access the ILL by going around and in front of the thick mass of the erectors.

After preparing and relaxing the outer layers of the low back and hip—including the erectors and the iliac crest region—use your thumbs together to slowly, gently sink into the area just anterior to the iliac crest, and just anterior to the mass of the erector muscles (Figure 3.3). This area will be sensitive or even ticklish on many people, so a slow, patient approach is imperative. Take your time, being mindful to take care for your thumbs by maintaining a small amount of flexion at each thumb joint. Stop and readjust your position, body use, pace, or direction (or do additional preparation) if the work is uncomfortable for either you or your client.

Once you've arrived at the lower "corner" of the space described by the iliac crest's juncture with the lumbars (Figure 3.4), pause and allow your client to relax even more. Small, active movements of your client's hip, or deep, slow breathing can facilitate the reduction in tonus, increased fascial elasticity, and proprioceptive refinement that are our goals. Patiently, gently, with minimal movement on your part, work both left and right iliolumbar ligaments.

See video of the Iliolumbar Ligament Technique at www.a-t.tv/v/pc06

Key points: Iliolumbar Ligament Technique

Indications include:
- Low- and mid-back pain, including pain referred to the hips, groin, rectum, genitals.
- Hip, sacroiliac, or hamstring pain.
- Low back stiffness or mobility restrictions.

Purpose
- Reduce any excessive tonus or over-participation of the muscles around the iliolumbar ligaments.
- Increased fascial differentiation and elasticity.

Instructions
With the client in a side lying position, and after preparing the outer layers of the low back and iliac crest:
1. Use two thumbs together just anterior to the iliac crest and the erectors. Slowly sink into the "corner" formed by the lumbars and the crest to find the Iliolumbar ligament.
2. Cue small active movements.
3. Work both sides.

Movements
- Slow, active hip flexion, extension, abduction, adduction, rotation.
- Slow, easy breathing.

Cautions
- Use caution with acute or unstable back conditions, including acute disc problems.

12th Rib Technique

Ida Rolf, the originator of Rolfing structural integration, placed special importance on freeing the 12th rib (6). As the posterior bony attachment of the diaphragm, and a stopover structure for many myofascial layers of the low back (including the TLF, Figure 3.5), the smallest pair of ribs plays an outsized role in posture, breathing, and back health.

Our aims in working with the 12th rib region are increased mobility, fascial elasticity, and proprioception. All of these are beneficial in and of themselves, and often result in less back pain. Although the 12th rib is a floating rib and so potentially quite mobile, when there is back pain, the rib is often sunk deep into dense, inelastic myofascial structures of the lower mid back. When these structures are structurally differentiated and proprioceptively awakened, people often experience increased fullness of breath, as well as freer, less painful movement of the back.

As the upper border of the lumbar space (the soft tissue region between the ribcage and pelvis), the 12th rib can be thought of as the complement or reflection of the iliac crest, which forms the lower margin of this same space. Starting far apart at their medial junctures with the spinal column, the 12th rib and iliac crest are much closer together at their lateral extremes. The distance between the end of the 12th rib and the iliac crest varies from person to person, affected by both the overall shape of the skeleton (such as torso length), and the elasticity of the TLF and the muscles it surrounds. When these soft tissues are denser and shorter, the distance between the rib end and the crest diminishes, and in some cases (such as with very short, compact waists or severe scoliosis) the rib can actually overlap the iliac crest and be found inside the pelvic bowl.

Left/right differences in this space's size can indicate spinal scoliosis or rib cage asymmetries, even when too mild to be otherwise noticeable. From a classical Rolfing and structural integration perspective, more distance and greater left/right evenness are generally considered desirable (7). We take a slightly different view in our Advanced Myofascial Techniques approach, where we emphasize evenness of mobility, elasticity, and body sense (proprioception) rather than focusing primarily on symmetrical

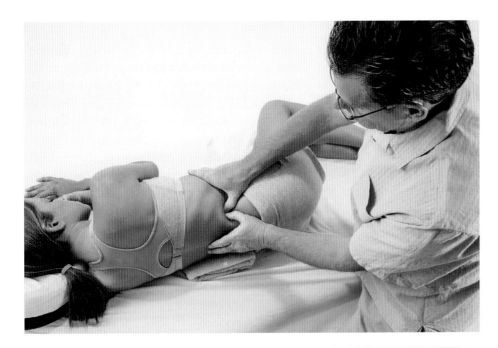

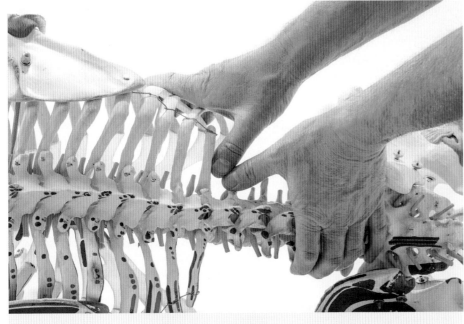

Figures 3.6/3.7

The 12th Rib Technique. After thorough preparation, use static pressure on the lower margin of the 12th rib, in combination with active client breathing, to increase tissue elasticity and rib mobility. Note that as with the Iliolumbar Ligament Technique, the approach is anterior to the erector group. Take care to avoid uncomfortable pressure directly on the rib's end or on the transverse processes.

distances, positions, or shapes. In my own clinical experience, symptoms such as back pain seem to correlate more clearly with mobility asymmetries than they do with positional asymmetries, and research findings support this (8). From this perspective, mild scoliosis or rib cage asymmetries are not necessarily problematic, unless there is pain or diminished function. Furthermore, these symptoms often respond more readily to our goals of improved tissue elasticity, mobility, and proprioception, than to changes in position alone.

As in the Iliac Crest Technique (Chapter 2), we'll focus on the soft tissue attachments to these bony structures. This will leverage the Golgi tendon organs' ability to modulate the resting tone of the entire muscular group (9). First, to reach the level of these osseous attachments, it is important to work down through the outer layers of the back's myofascia, including the superficial fascia, the serratus posterior inferior, the outer layers of the thoracolumbar fascia, and the muscular tissue of the erectors, as we did in the Thoracolumbar Fascia Technique in the previous chapter.

Once you've prepared these outer structures, carefully locate the sensitive end of the 12th rib. While meticulously avoiding pressure directly against this rib's end (or into the free end of the 11th rib just lateral and superior to it), use your thumbs to apply gentle pressure to the 12th rib's inferior margin (Figures 3.6 and 3.7). It is on this lower edge of the rib's shaft that most of the back's tissue layers attach. If the rib is difficult to distinguish, or seems deeply embedded within the back's tissue layers, additional preparation may be needed.

Once on the rib's lower margin, ask for full, gentle breath in order to facilitate fascial softening, and to increase proprioceptive awareness of this often-forgotten region. Keep your pressure directed superiorly into the lower margin of the rib, staying right on the bone, in order to avoid pressing into the organs or the lumbar transverse processes. You'll sometimes feel thicker, hardened tissue along this bony margin; these are the attachments of the TLF. Wait in each place for a tissue response; then proceed medially and superiorly, pausing in each place to facilitate increased elasticity and awareness.

The lateral arcuate ligament is a thickening in the most anterior layer of the TLF, similar to the iliolumbar ligament at its lower attachment, in this case just anterior to the 12th rib. Although it is probably too small and too far anterior to be directly palpated, your work to free the 12th rib's mobility will indirectly affect this ligament as well.

Key points: 12th Rib Technique

Indications include:

- Restricted posterior motion of the diaphragm in breathing.
- Restricted or painful movement of the back, including flexion, sidebending, rotation, breathing, etc.

Purpose

- Increased options for breath mobility in the back.
- Increased proprioceptive refinement, especially related to breath and standing.

Instructions

With the client in a side lying position and after preparing the outer fascial layers:

1. Carefully apply pressure to the inferior margin of the 12th rib using thumbs.
2. Wait with static pressure combined with client's breath for a Golgi tendon response.
3. Once mobility increases and tissues soften, move to a new portion of the 12th rib and repeat.

Movements

- Full, gentle breathing.

Summary

These two techniques work the dense, ligamentous parts of the thoracolumbar fascia at the upper and lower extremes of the lumbar space. As with the TLF in our last column, using these two techniques on acute or unstable back conditions, including acute disc problems, is contraindicated in most cases, at least until you have gained a considerable amount of experience in their application, and are very familiar with how your individual client responds to direct work.

Applied correctly, these techniques are quite safe, and you'll see obvious and gratifying results with most mild to moderate low back pain. Although preparation, sensitivity, patience, rapport, and skill are each important when working at these deep levels, the often dramatic improvements in mobility and comfort of the low back will make it very worth the effort.

References

[1] Vleeming, A. et al. (2007) *Lumbopelvic Pain*. Edinburgh: Elsevier. p. 64–73.

[2] Langevin, H.M. et al. (2009) Ultrasound evidence of altered lumbar connective tissue structure in human subjects with chronic low back pain. *BMC Musculoskeletal Disorders*. 10. p. 151.

[3] Stecco, A. et al. (2013) Ultrasonography in myofascial neck pain: Randomized clinical trial for diagnosis and follow-up. *Surgical and Radiologic Anatomy*. (August 23). doi: 10.1007/s00276-013-1185-2.

[4] Travell, J.G. and Simons, D.G. (1998) *Myofascial Pain and Dysfunction: The Trigger Point Manual*. Vol. 2: *The Lower Extremities*. Lippincott Williams & Wilkins.

[5] Maigne, J.Y. and Maigne, R. (1991) Trigger point of the posterior iliac crest: Painful iliolumbar ligament insertion or cutaneous dorsal ramus pain? An anatomic study. *Archives of Physical Medicine and Rehabilitation*. 72(10). p. 734–737.

[6] Rolf, I.P. IPR Audio Files, Tape A2. 8:50. http://www.rolfguild.org/av/rolfa2.html. [Accessed December 2015]

[7] Rolf, I.P. IPR Audio Files, Tape A2. 13:00. http://www.rolfguild.org/av/rolfa2.html. [Accessed December 2015]

[8] Lee, D. (2004) *The Pelvic Girdle. 3rd ed.* Churchill Livingstone.

[9] Schleip,R. (2003) Fascial plasticity: A new neurobiological explanation, Part I. *Journal of Bodywork and Movement Therapies*. 7(1). p. 14.

Picture credits

Figures 3.1, 3.2, and 3.5 Primal Pictures, used by permission.
Figures 3.3, 3.4, 3.6, and 3.7 Advanced-Trainings.com.

Study Guide

The Iliolumbar Ligament & 12th Rib

1 **Along with thoracolumbar fascia (TLF) thickening, what does this chapter cite as another factor in low back pain?**

a TFL hypermobility
b TLF layer immobility
c TFL thinness
d TLF weakness

2 **Where are the iliolumbar ligaments?**

a anterior to the erector spinae
b anterior to the 12th rib
c posterior to the erector spinae
d embedded within the erector spinae

3 **The chapter says that mild scoliosis and rib asymmetries can be considered problematic when:**

a there are also shoulder girdle asymmetries
b they have been diagnosed by an physician
c there is pain
d there are clearly visible shape asymmetries

4 **What direction of pressure does the chapter suggest the practitioner use when working on the 12th rib?**

a superior
b inferior
c medial
d anterior

5 **What active movement does the text recommend for facilitating 12th rib work?**

a full gentle breath
b deep, focused breath
c hip flexion and extension
d belly extension

For Answer Keys, visit www.Advanced-Trainings.com/v2key/

The Mesentery and Abdomen

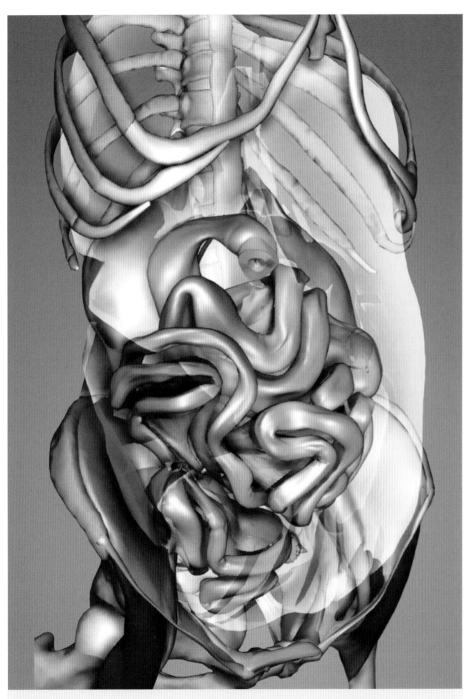

Figure 4.1

The mesentery (blue) forms the fascial connection between the intestines and the posterior abdominal fascia on the front of the spine. It provides both support and a pathway for the viscera's neural complex. Pictured here is the mesentery of the small intestines, and the parietal peritoneum (transparent blue), which is continuous with it.

Have you ever had a gut feeling? A sense of knowing something, without knowing *how* you knew? As body-oriented practitioners, we might wonder: why is this called a "gut" feeling, anyway?

An instinctual sense of certainty has long been associated with our bellies, and not just in the English-speaking world. The French also say this kind of knowing is *viscéral*, the Japanese speak of *hara-gei* (1), and the German use *Bauchgefühl* (literally, a belly feeling).

Along with instinctual certainty, the gut is associated with many other body-mind phenomena. Why do we say our stomach gets "tied up in knots" by stress? We don't say we have "butterflies in the arm" when we're excited or anxious—why are the butterflies in the stomach? Along with the heart, the belly is probably more often linked to emotional, mental, and psychological states than any other part of the body. Understanding the significant role of the viscera in the body's emotional responses can only help manual therapists in their work.

It has long been known that hands-on work with the abdomen can influence emotional states as well. For example, in the 1930s the Austrian neuropsychiatrist Wilhelm Reich used deep, often painful massage on the abdomen (and elsewhere) to break up the muscular tension he saw as "armoring" against the free flow of emotion. Combined with deep, full breathing, his abdominal manipulation produced strong emotional responses in his patients (2). Though his emotionally evocative methods were (and remain) controversial, his ideas about the role of bodily tension in emotional health profoundly influenced generations of body-oriented therapists such as Fritz Perls, Alexander Lowen, Ida Rolf, and many others (3 and 4).

In contrast to a painfully evocative, armor- busting approach, gentle, non-invasive work with the abdomen can be calming, quieting, and deeply comforting. Moreover, skilled and sensitive work with the abdomen's fascial structures can provide non-invasive ways to address a surprisingly long list of client complaints affecting both body and mind (see "Indications" later in this chapter).

The enteric nervous system

The viscera's complex neurology might help explain why we associate so many body-mind phenomena with this part of the body, and why hands-on work here can be either emotionally settling, or emotionally evocative. The enteric nervous system, our viscera's neural network, contains some 100 million neurons, more than either the spinal cord or the rest of the peripheral nervous system (5). The enteric system also uses over 30 neurotransmitters, more than anywhere outside the central nervous system (6). In fact, more than 95 percent of the body's serotonin is found in the gut, which is one reason why drugs that alter this neurotransmitter's balance, such as some antidepressants, can also cause gastric disturbances (and why osteoporosis may be affected by the viscera, since serotonin regulates bone density).

The size and intricacy of the belly's enteric nervous system have led some science writers to call it the "second brain" (7). Though not capable of truly brain-like thought (8), the enteric nervous system is far more complicated than what is required for digestive functions alone. It also seems to contribute a great deal to our ongoing emotional state, sending information to the brain where it constantly informs our felt sense of ourselves, as a kind of predisposition or background mood for the brain's mental processes (9).

Neurologically, the digestive viscera are innervated by the dorsal branch of the vagus nerve—a key part of the parasympathetic nervous system. It is the parasympathetic "rest-and-repair" system that calms and regulates the sympathetic "fight or flight" activation of stress, fear, and trauma. The relaxed, sleepy feeling after a meal is an example of the vagus nerve at work.

Because the vagus nerve's axons are about 80 percent sensory (that is, carrying information from the viscera up to the brain), our gut affects our brain much more than the brain affects the gut. This might be why hands-on work with the abdomen seems particularly sedative, at least when done non-invasively and gently. Skilled work with the belly can literally, and very effectively, calm an upset mind.

A more extreme version of this calming effect may be involved in stronger trauma responses, as well. When the nervous system perceives a threat to survival, the dorsal branch of the vagus nerve is thought to trigger the fainting, passing out, dissociation, or loss of bowel control that can sometimes result from a strong shock, threat, or trauma (10).

The mesentery's mysterious anatomy

The intestines are suspended in the abdominal cavity by the mesentery, a folded fascial membrane (Figure 4.1) connected to the anterior aspect of the lumbar region. As well as providing structural support for the intestines, the mesentery encases the many nerves and rich vasculature of the digestive tract (Figure 4.2).

Our understanding of the mesentery's anatomy has changed dramatically as result of a large-scale prospective study of mesenteric anatomy in 2012, the first to study the mesentery's changes over time (11). Classically, most anatomy texts described the mesentery

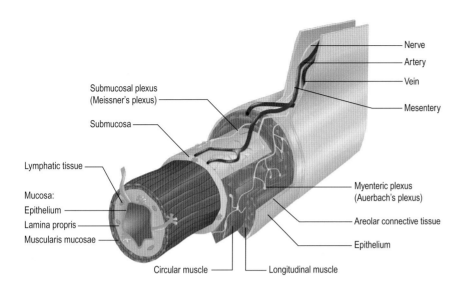

Figure 4.2

The mesentery's tissue layers surround the intestines along their entire 18–25 foot length, and encase their rich vasculature and complex neural network.

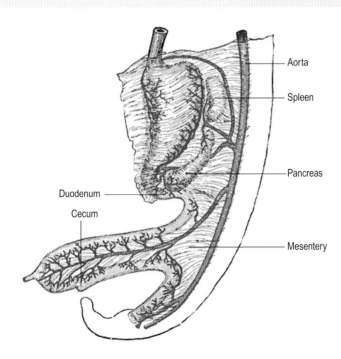

Figure 4.3

The developing mesentery (blue) in a human embryo of 6 weeks, showing a simpler schema of the mesentery's role in supporting the digestive tract and its neurovasculature from the anterior aspect of the emerging vertebral column.

in the embryo as a single structure connecting the emerging viscera to the notochord (the precursor to the spinal column, Figure 4.3), which then split in adulthood into a convoluted collection of several separate fascial units (namely, the mesentery of the small intestine; the left, right, the transverse mesocolon; and the mesoappendix, mesosigmoid and mesorectum). The 2012 study revealed a much simpler anatomy, and confirmed what many surgeons had long observed: that the mesentery remains unified in almost all adults, and that the previously described segments are just features of a single integrated structure that supports the intestines along their entire 18- to 27-foot length, from their start near the stomach, to their terminus at the rectum. This large, combined structure is referred to as the mesenteric organ, or simply the *mesentery*.

Even with this simplification, the mesentery's anatomy can be difficult to visualize. Picture a weighted fishing net hanging from its center (Figure 4.4): the intestines would be analogous to the weights around the net's periphery, with the mesenteric root (Figures 4.5 and 4.6) being the net's point of suspension on the front side of the low back.

It is because of the mesentery's attachment to the fascia anterior of the lumbars that the pull of the intestines' weight can be implicated in low back pain.

The mesentery is itself part of a larger fascial continuity that includes the parietal peritoneum, a sac of thin, resilient fascia that surrounds the abdominal viscera (Figure 4.7). To expand our hanging-net analogy, not only does the mesenteric "net" hang from the posterior abdominal wall, it is also continuous with a net (the peritoneum) that covers the wall, and lines the entire room (Figure 4.8).

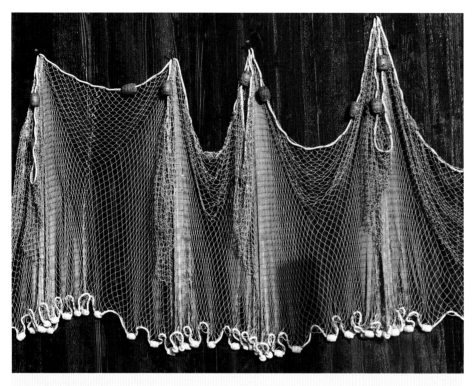

Figure 4.4

The mesentery's anatomy is analogous to a weighted net, suspended from the mesenteric root.

The Mesentery Technique

The abdomen is a very personal and sensitive part of the body. This is possibly related to body image (habitual tensing of the abdomen or holding the belly in), to the body-mind dimensions we mentioned earlier, or to the fact that our abdomens are rarely touched by others outside of very intimate contexts. For these reasons, working with the abdomen is appropriate only when rapport and good client-practitioner communication have already been established.

Fortunately, the complexities of the belly's nervous system, fascial anatomy, and interpersonal dimensions are all balanced by the extreme simplicity of the technique itself.

Rolling the peritoneal bubble

With your client on her side, gently cradle the abdominal contents, one hand in the space between the pelvis and the ribcage, and the other on the upper lumbars, behind the mesenteric root (Figure 4.9).

Your intention at this stage is simply to support and ease the organs encased in the peritoneal sac. The type of touch required is different than the touch used for other purposes. We are not trying to release or stretch the fascia; nor are we massaging the viscera. Because of its very sophisticated, sensitive neurology, and its looser, softer tissues, the belly responds well to very light, patient, and perceptive touch. Your client's enteric nervous system is sensing you, perhaps even more than you're sensing it. With this in mind, hold the peritoneum as if you were holding a large, delicate, sentient soap bubble (Figure 4.10).

Before moving or manipulating, let your client become accustomed to your touch. You might invite a slow, full inhalation into the belly, and an even slower, easy exhalation (which gently activates a parasympathetic response). With-

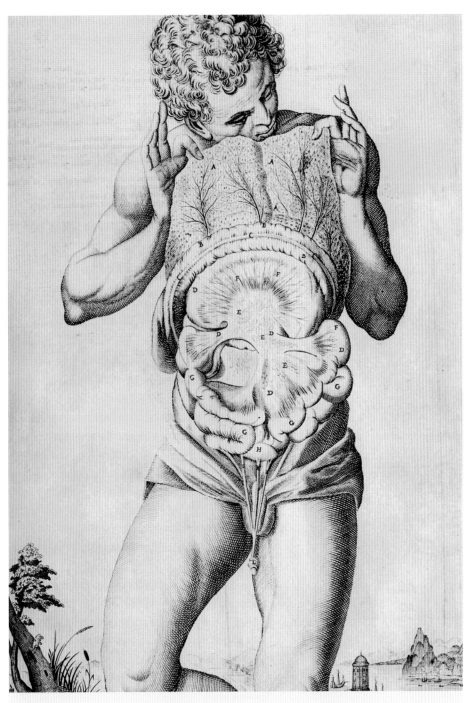

Figure 4.5
The mesentery's root (labeled E) from an 1627 engraving from Giulio Casserio's *Tabulae Anatomicae*.

out stressing, stretching, or bursting the metaphorical soap bubble, begin to gently roll the visceral sac in various directions: medially up off the table, cranially toward the head, and so on, all in super-slow motion. Your hand remains soft, without sliding, poking, or exerting effort (Figure 4.11). Your intention is gentle, whole-abdomen mobilization and relaxation. Working with the breath, monitor your client's ability to rest and let you support the weight of her viscera. If you feel your client tensing or holding the breath, stop or back up, and invite your client to relax the belly even more.

Easing the mesenteric net

In the same patient, sensitive manner, you can now feel for the mesentery itself. It is important to emphasize that we are not trying to touch the mesentery directly, nor are we using direct technique to stretch or lengthen it. Because of the belly's extreme sensitivity, we use indirect technique here, slackening rather than stretching the mesenteric tissues, by gently supporting the abdominal contents cranially (toward the head) and medially (toward the midline) in the direction of the mesenteric root.

We can be a bit more direct than we were with the soap-bubble peritoneum, but still very delicate and soft in our touch. Moving the abdominal contents in this way is much like moving water balloons in a tub (Figure 4.12)—the viscera have the same kind of delicate, slippery, fluid-filled qualities as water balloons, and your touch should take this into account.

On a client with a smaller belly (Figure 4.11), a light touch is all that is needed. On a person with a larger gut, we can use some strength to take the actual weight of the viscera, and relieve the mesentery's pull on the spine. In both cases, as you support the intestines toward the mesenteric root, feel for a gentle easing in the lumbars with your posterior hand. This may take the duration

See video of
the Mesentery
Technique at
www.a-t.tv/sb03

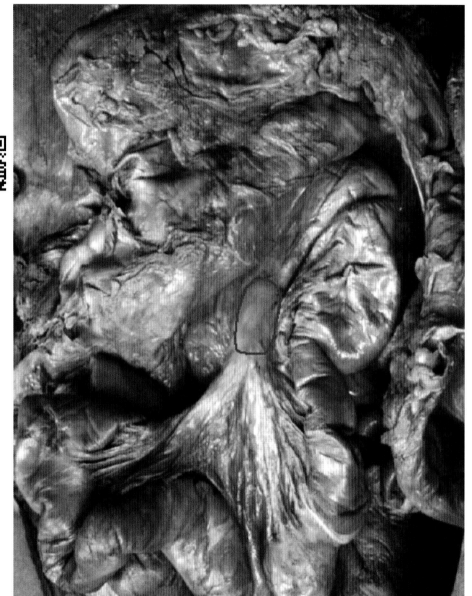

Figure 4.6

The mesenteric root (circled in red) on the front of the lumbar spine is revealed here by pulling the large and small intestines aside.

of several breaths, and will be most apparent when there is mesenteric involvement in low back lordosis or discomfort.

Wait for this easing of the posterior hand; or for a quieting of the breathing rhythm; or other signs of autonomic nervous system shift, such as a sigh,

Key points: The Mesentery Technique

Indications include:
- Digestive distress, irritable bowel syndrome.
- Low back pain, disc issues, and axial sciatic pain.
- Pregnancy and postpartum recovery.
- Abdominal surgery and injury recovery.
- Osteoporosis.
- Sacroiliac joint pain.
- Stress, depression, anxiety or unresolved trauma.

Purpose
- Ease mobility or tissue restrictions affecting the viscera.
- Ease tension or pain in the low back, SI joint, or lumbar nerve roots via the mesenteric root.
- Refine awareness (interoception) of abdominal sensation.
- Calm ANS activation via the enteric nervous system.

Instructions
Be sure to establish rapport, explain the purpose, and get overt permission before working with the abdomen:
1. In side lying position, gently cradle the abdominal contents while supporting the lumbars with the other hand.
2. Wait for client to surrender the weight of the organs into your supporting hand, and for the low back to ease.
3. Then, as if moving a soap bubble, begin to gently, slowly roll the visceral sac, feeling for mobility in various directions.
4. Wait for breath motion to free any restrictions found.

Movements
Use your client's breath; with a slight emphasis on lengthening the exhalation.

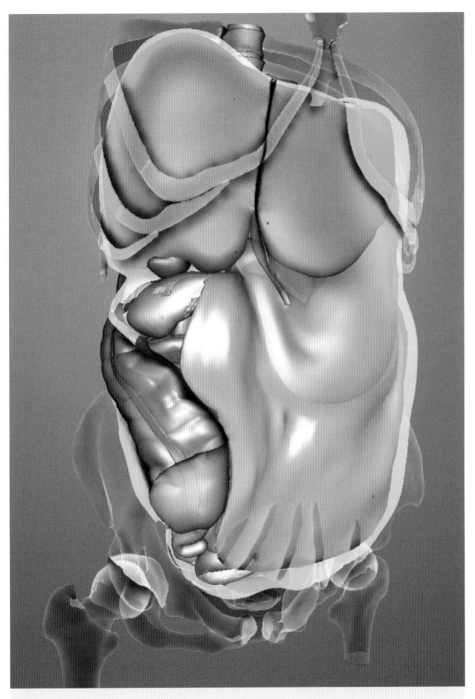

Figure 4.7
The parietal peritoneum (blue) is a thin, resilient fascial layer surrounding the intestines and lining the abdominal cavity.

twitch, or eye flutter. Then, slowly release the hold. Repeat this support of the mesentery and waiting for a response in various directions; then, continue with other aspects of your treatment.

Indications

The mesentery, as the structural connector of the spine, intestines, and the neural complexes associated with both, can be thought of as a key access route for working with a variety of client complaints. Consider including the Mesentery Technique when working with the following client conditions, amongst others:

- **Digestive distress, irritable bowel syndrome, and related gastric complaints.** The potential mechanical effects on the intestines; the interoceptive (sensory) refinement from the focused attention of hands-on work; and, especially, the calming effects of touch itself, can all have beneficial effects on intestinal and digestive complaints.
- **Low back pain, disc issues, and axial sciatic pain,** due to the mechanical pull of the mesenteric root on the anterior lumbars, especially in obesity. (For a discussion of axial vs. versus appendicular sciatica, see *Advanced Myofascial Techniques, Volume I*, p 107–109).
- **Pregnancy and post-partum recovery.** Peritoneal and mesenteric work can help ease displaced and crowded viscera.
- **Recovery from abdominal surgeries and injuries.** Gentle manipulation has been shown to reduce adhesions and inflammation of the abdominal fascia, and improve post-operative intestinal functioning (12).
- **Osteoporosis.** Serotonin has a regulatory effect on bone density (13).
- **Sacroiliac (SI) joint pain,** particularly of the right-side SI joint, as the slightly diagonal mesenteric root crosses the anterior aspect of the right sacroiliac joint [endnote 14].

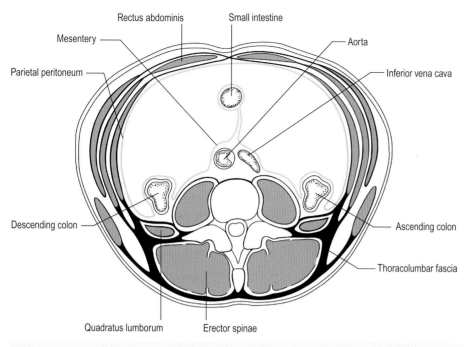

Figure 4.8

Schematic cross-section of the lumbar region, showing the continuity of the mesentery and the parietal peritoneum (both in blue) and their relationship to the spine.

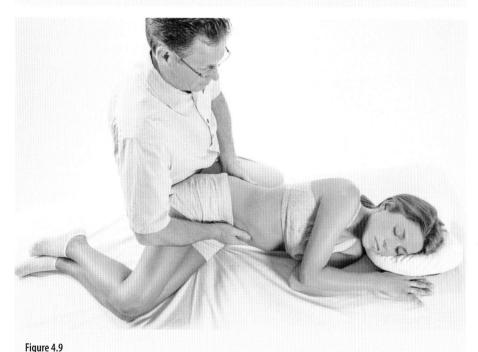

Figure 4.9

The Mesentery Technique, part one: supporting the visceral sac of the peritoneum. Sensitive, patient motion testing of the entire peritoneal sac increases ease and gentle mobility.

- **Stress, depression, anxiety, and the effects of unresolved trauma,** due to the enteric nervous system's role in regulating serotonin levels, as well as the role of the parasympathetic nervous system and the vagus nerve in the body's responses to trauma.

We should clarify that although the peritoneum and mesentery are visceral connective tissue structures, the technique applied here is not Visceral Manipulation Therapy, the method developed by French osteopath Jean-Pierre Barral. Practitioners and teachers of his sophisticated system of subtle organ manipulation emphasize caution and sensitivity, and warn against untrained attempts at organ manipulation (15). Caution when working with the sensitive viscera is very justified, as would be referral to a trained psychotherapist for depression or unresolved trauma, or a physician whenever medical conditions are suspected.

What are we accomplishing?

If we aren't trying to stretch fascia, or massage organs, what are we accomplishing with such a gentle, indirect technique?

Keep in mind the "second brain" nature of the gut. If you could directly manipulate the brain itself, you probably wouldn't try to mechanically stretch or soften its tissues. Your simple touch itself would have profound effects, based on quieting and calming, awakening sensation, and inviting ease.

However, a gentle touch, such as we're using here, can have surprisingly tangible effects on tissue as well. A 2012 Medline-listed study of surgery-induced abdominal adhesions in rats showed that gentle abdominal massage, performed only to a depth that "did not elicit flinching or biting" by the rat subjects, reduced and prevented fascial adhesions in the gut, as well as decreased intraperitoneal inflammation and helped restore post-operative intestinal propulsion (ileus). Interestingly, the investigators noted that during manipulation "the rats became calm and allowed deep palpation" (16), which would come as no surprise when we remember the viscera's role in parasympathetic responses.

As you experiment with these gentle mesentery techniques in your practice, keep in mind you're affecting both the tissues of the body, and the processes of the nervous system, across the entire body-mind spectrum.

References

[1] Hodgson, J.D., Sano, Y., and Graham, J.L. (2008) *Doing Business with the New Japan: Succeeding in America's Richest International Market*. Lanham, MD: Rowman & Littlefield Publishers. p. 238.

[2] Reich, P. (1989) *Book of Dreams*. Dutton Obelisk.

[3] Bocian, B. (2010) *Fritz Perls in Berlin 1893–1933*. Peter Hammer Verlag GmbH.

[4] Jacobsen, E. (2011) Structural integration: Origins and development. *Journal of Alternative and Complementary Medicine*. 17(9). p. 775–780.

[5] Gershon, M.D. (1998) *The Second Brain: The Scientific Basis of Gut Instinct and a Groundbreaking New Understanding of Nervous Disorders of the Stomach and Intestines*. Harper.

[6] Gershon, M.D. (1998) ibid.

[7] Gershon, M.D. (1998) ibid.

[8] Mayer, E. (2010), Professor of Physiology, Psychiatry, and Biobehavioral Sciences at the David Geffen School of Medicine at UCLA, as quoted in Adam Hadhazy, Think twice: How the gut's 'Second Brain' influences mood and well-being, *Scientific American*. http://www.scientificamerican.com/article/gut-second-brain/. [Accessed December 2015]

[9] Hadhazy, A. (2010) ibid.

[10] Porges, S.W. (2011) *The Polyvagal Theory: Neurophysiological Foundations of Emotions, Attachment, Communication, and Self-regulation*. New York: WW Norton.

[11] Culligan, K., Coffey, J.C., Kiran, R.P., Kalady, M., Lavery, I.C., and Remzi, F.H. (April 2012) The mesocolon: A prospective observational study. *Colorectal Disease*. 14(4). p. 421–428; discussion p. 428–430.

[12] Bove, G.M. and Chapelle, S.L. (2012) Visceral mobilization can lyse and prevent peritoneal adhesions in a rat model. *Journal of Bodywork and Movement Therapies*. 16(1). p. 76–82.

[13] Yadav, V.K. et al. (2010) Pharmacological inhibition of gut-derived serotonin synthesis is a potential bone anabolic treatment for osteoporosis. *Nature Medicine*. 16. p. 308–312.

[14] Burch, J.P. (2001) Core balance: Interdisciplinary Structural Integration. *Massage & Bodywork* April/May. p. 22–31.

[15] Barral, J.-P. and Mercier, P. (2000) *Visceral Manipulation*. Revised ed. Seattle, WA: Eastland Press.

[16] Bove, G.M. ibid.

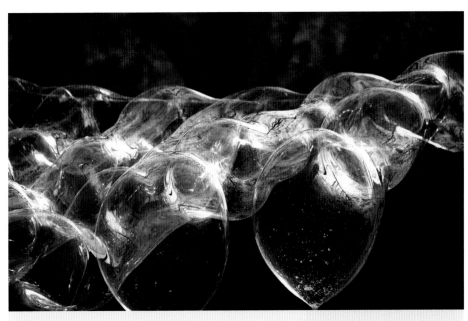

Figure 4.10

The perceptive, gentle touch needed for the Mesentery Technique is analogous to lightly holding a soap bubble.

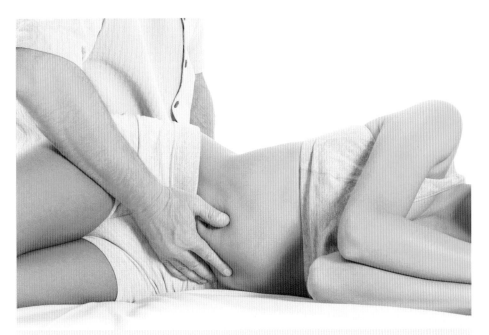

Figure 4.11

The Mesentery Technique, part two: gently support the weight of the viscera, and lift the intestines slightly toward the mesenteric root. The posterior hand feels for a subtle softening or easing in the lumbar spine at the level of the mesenteric root.

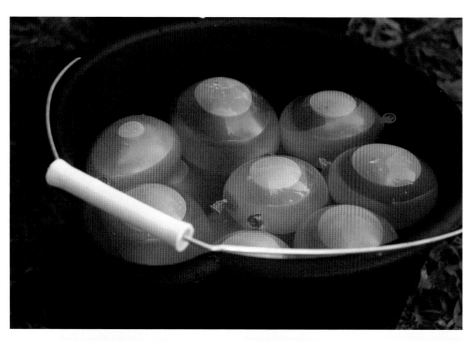

Figure 4.12

The abdominal viscera have the same kind of delicate, slippery, fluid-filled qualities as water balloons in a tub; your touch should take this into account.

Picture credits

Figures 4.1, 4.6, and 4.7 Primal Pictures, used by permission.

Figure 4.2 Göran Jönsson, used under CCA-SA 3.0.

Figure 4.3 Grey's Anatomy of the Human Body, 1918. Image is in the public domain.

Figures 4.4, 4.10, and 4.12 Thinkstock.

Figure 4.5 from Giulio Casserio's *Tabulae anatomicae*, 1627. Artist: Francesco Valesio. Image is in the public domain.

Figures 4.8, 4.9, and 4.11 Advanced-Trainings.com.

Study Guide

The Mesentery and the Abdomen

1 Because of its attachment site, the text states that the mesentery can be directly involved in which symptom?

a hiccups
b low back pain
c stomach ache
d pelvic floor pain

2 What is the stated goal of the "Rolling the Peritoneal Bubble" step of the Mesentery Technique?

a to stimulate the smooth muscles of the intestines
b to manually release gas bubbles caught within the abdominal contents
c to massage the viscera
d to mobilize the peritoneal sac

3 Which statement best describes the enteric nervous system?

a it is another term for the parasympathetic nervous system
b it is the dorsal branch of the vagus nerve
c it is the complex neural network of the viscera
d it is another term for the entire nervous system

4 Because of its sensitive, sophisticated neurology, what kind of touch is recommended for these techniques?

a slow, firm, and deep touch
b light, patient, and perceptive touch
c light, superficial, and brief touch
d two-handed, rhythmic, and intentional touch

5 What is the stated goal of the "Easing the Mesenteric Net" step of the Mesentery Technique?

a to ease the lumbar spine by lifting the mesentery towards the spine
b to ease the respiratory diaphragm by lifting the mesentery towards the head
c to differentiate and increase elasticity of the mesentery's fascial folds
d to prepare the viscera for deeper and more direct work

For Answer Keys, visit www.Advanced-Trainings.com/v2key/

The psoas is a true celebrity. In terms of the attention it gets, and the claims made for it, the psoas has superstar-status in fields as diverse as yoga, massage, physical therapy, Pilates, chiropractic, strengthening and conditioning, martial arts, as well as structural integration and Rolfing. Like other famous stars, the life-story of the psoas is probably a mixture of fact and fiction, where speculation, mystery, hyperbole, and controversy have blended with the psoas' truly special qualities, eccentricities, and abilities.

Hidden away deep in the abdomen where its workings are more hidden than other, more superficial muscles, the psoas is the subject of numerous (and often contradictory) theories, rumors, and assertions. Rightly or wrongly, some of the many claims about the psoas are that it is:

- The deepest muscle in the body.
- The only muscle to connect the legs with the spine.
- Along with the tongue, the most sensitive muscle in the body (1).
- The strongest hip flexor (2) or, not a hip flexor at all (3).
- A lateral rotator of the hip (4); or, a medial rotator of the hip (5) or, not a rotator of the hip (6).
- Able to deepen the lumbar curve by contracting (7); or, able to *flatten* the lumbar curve by contracting (8) or, not related to lumbar curve (9).
- Involved in most back pain (10) or, not particularly relevant to back pain (11).
- "Just another spinal muscle" (12) or, it is the "muscle of the soul"(13).
- Important to work directly (14) or, should never be worked directly (15) or, is physically impossible to work directly (16).

Controversy

From this list, we can see that there is quite a bit of debate about the psoas' biomechanical function. But another thing is also clear: direct myofascial work with the psoas is itself controversial. It is easy to find heated online and social-media debates about the effectiveness, methods, or advisability of psoas work; some of these exchanges have even spurred threats of legal action (17).

Rather than trying to argue here for which parts of the psoas' divisive, larger-than-life reputation might be either true or false, I'll make some simple and practical suggestions for working with the psoas.[1] My suggestions are not necessarily scientific or research-based, as much as they are empirical: that is, they are based on my own clinical, teaching, and supervising experience. And though admittedly biased by my own training, style, and proclivities, my views are tempered by my interested reading and study of many others' reports, opinions, and approaches.

But first, let's review some anatomy.

Psoas anatomy

The term "psoas" is usually shorthand for the *psoas major*, a pair of layered fusiform (long and narrow) unipennate (having short oblique fibers) muscles deep in the abdomen. The psoas' posterior layer attaches to the transverse processes of the five lumbar vertebrae, and its anterior layer to the lateral aspects of the vertebral bodies and intervertebral discs of T12-L5. The psoas major joins with the iliacus muscle in a common tendon at the lesser trochanter of the femur to form the iliopsoas complex, which is surrounded by the thin, tough iliac fascia (Figure 5.1). (In about 50 percent of people,

---

1 For a thorough and well-reasoned overview of the differing views of the psoas major's biomechanics, see Muscolino, J. "Psoas Major Function" in MTJ, Body Mechanics column, Spring 2013. 17–31.

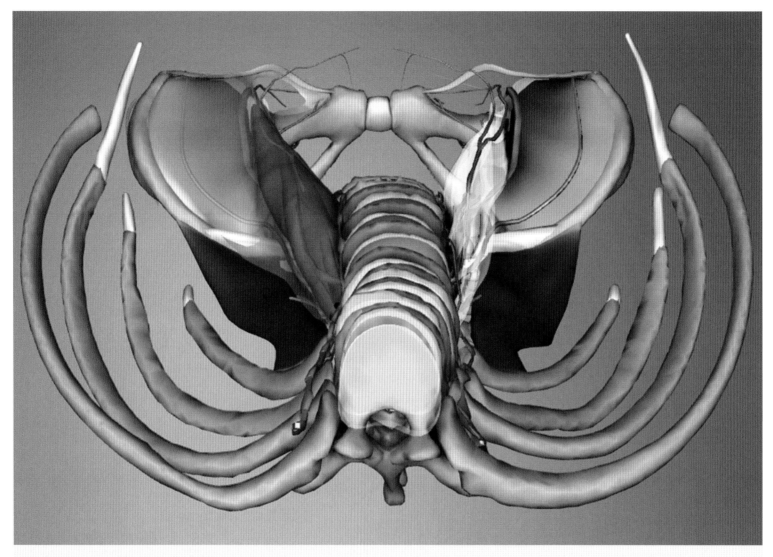

Figure 5.1

The psoas major muscles (green), from above. The surrounding iliac fascia is visible on the left; the transparency of the right psoas muscle reveals the lumbar plexus' nerves within the belly of the psoas major, which contribute to the psoas' extreme sensitivity.

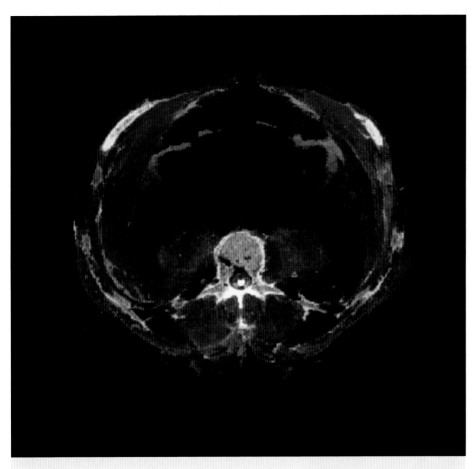

Figure 5.2

The psoas and the spinal erectors arrayed around the lumbar spine, like four guy-wires stabilizing a mast.

a smaller, parallel, and partially separate *psoas minor* muscle is also present, which terminates by attaching to the iliac fascia and the inside of the pelvic bowl.)

The left and right psoas, together with the left and right spinal erector groups, are arrayed around the spinal column like four guy wires around a mast (Figure 5.2). In sitting or standing, the right and left psoas work bilaterally to stabilize the vertical spine. In sidebending and twisting, they work unilaterally to exert powerful torques on the spine. Because of their role in twisting the trunk, surgically severing the "short" psoas was at one time thought to improve severe scoliosis, until this extreme measure was thankfully deemed ineffective (18) (which also suggests that although it rotates the trunk, psoas contraction is not a primary cause of idiopathic scoliosis).

The psoas is extremely sensitive. This is likely related to its proprioceptive function in upright postures. If we think of the psoas as a proprioceptive sensor, sending information about spinal position and movement to the central nervous system, rather than solely as a motoric muscle, it'll help us approach it with the sensitivity and subtlety it needs.

The psoas' sensitivity is in part due to the numerous nerves that pass around, within, and through its muscle mass (Figure 5.3). Lying right alongside the spinal nerve exits, the psoas' front and back layers sandwich the nerves of the lumbar plexus (Figure 5.4). These nerve trunks, which give rise to the obturator, genitofemoral, sciatic, and other nerves, pass right though the psoas' belly. This unique anatomy gives the psoas a potential role in certain types of nerve entrapment pain, such as groin pain, sciatic pain, or femoral nerve pain (19). In my own practice, I have observed a clear improvement in many clients' axial sciatic pain after careful work with and around the psoas (see *Advanced Myofascial Techniques, Volume I*, Sciatic Pain).

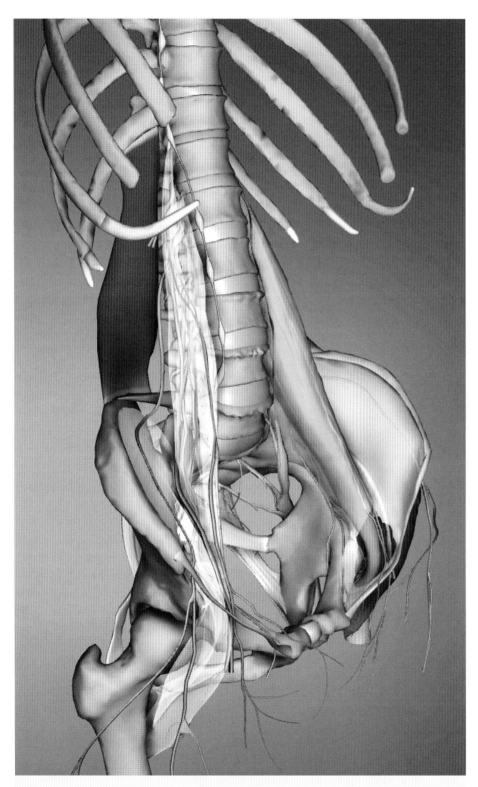

Figure 5.3
The psoas major (green) and the nerves that pass through its belly. The quadratus lumborum is also shown (red).

Is psoas work safe?

Most of the critics of direct manual therapy with the psoas are concerned about the risk of internal damage from rough manipulation of the psoas. They do have a point—the psoas is indeed surrounded by structures that are more delicate than the muscles and dense connective tissue that most bodyworkers are accustomed to working, stretching, and "releasing." These sensitive structures include the many nerves and plexi that surround and invest the psoas muscles; the aorta and inferior vena cava; the kidneys, their ducts, and their vasculature; the ureters, ovaries, fallopian tubes, and uterus; the abdominal lymph vessels and nodes; and of course the intestines and their supporting mesentery. Without a doubt, insensitive, painful, or strong work around these delicate structures of the abdomen is very ill-advised, and could be dangerous. Fortunately, injuries from psoas work seem very rare. My reasonably extensive Internet searches found just one account of client injury associated with myofascial, massage, structural integration, manual therapy, or physical therapy psoas techniques. That single report was an uninvolved party's social media account of a practitioner apparently "stepping on" a client's psoas (20). In spite of the relative rarity of these complaints, or the extreme nature of this single example, the potential for client injury from insensitive abdominal work is probably very real.

But strong pressure is rarely (if ever) needed in our approach to the psoas—its delicate, proprioceptive nature means it responds quickly and easily to gentle touch; and this gentle touch, especially when used with the necessary sensitivity and communication with the client, is (in my opinion and experience) very unlikely to damage or disrupt the surrounding structures.

Some writers (Koch in particular) are concerned about potentially upsetting emotional responses

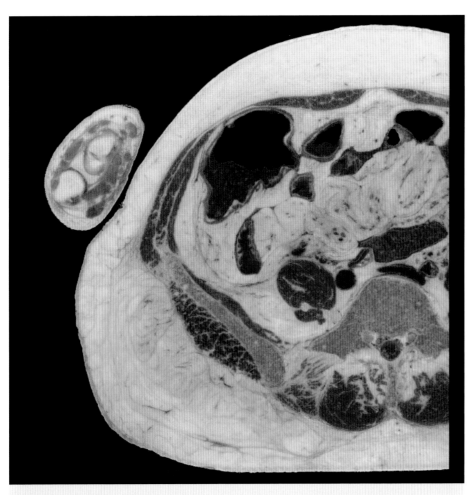

Figure 5.4

The ventral rami of the third and fourth lumbar spinal nerves (green) sandwiched between the anterior and posterior layers of the psoas major.

to psoas work. It is true that abdominal work, no matter how gentle, can sometimes elicit emotional responses from clients, with sadness, anxiousness, or other feelings sometimes arising as the belly softens. Though these emotions can appear during work elsewhere in the body too, there does seem to be a special role in the body-mind continuum for the abdomen, and perhaps for the psoas in particular. This might be related to the role of the belly's enteric nervous system (parts of which pass through and around the psoas) in setting the emotional background to our state of mind (as discussed in Chapter 4, *The Mesentery and the Abdomen*). Interestingly, somatic body-mind methodologies have long included work with the abdomen and psoas. In the 1930s, 40s, and 50s, Austrian psychiatrist and body-therapy pioneer Wilhelm Reich used deep (and often painful) abdominal massage to "break up" the muscular tension as a part of his body-mind treatments; one of his indicators of somato-emotional health was the free, easy movement of the belly in breathing (21). Reich's work gave rise to Alexander Lowen's Bioenergetics in the 1970s, which used stress positions and deep breathing along with physical manipulation (22). In the 1980s, Feldenkrais-trained Thomas Hannah described the psoas' involvement in the body's "red light" reflexes of protective flexion in response to unpleasant stimuli (23). More recently, bodyworker and trauma-therapy writer David Berceli has asserted that the psoas contracts involuntarily in response to trauma or alarm, as an automatic part of the body's instinctive crouching and protective reflexes. He asserts that these contractions can accumulate until "released" (by stress positions and trembling, in his method) (24).

These examples do suggest that extra sensitivity to the client's internal experience is especially important in hands-on work with the belly and psoas. Very occasionally, emotions surface, as they sometimes do with hands-on work elsewhere in the body. When the practitioner affords these client responses respect, gentle acknowledgement, and a bit of time, these feelings typically resolve on their own, often leaving a sense of lightness and well-being once they have passed.

In our Advanced Myofascial Techniques trainings, we include gentle, direct work with the psoas in our technique repertory, as we have seen clear benefits from working here that are not easily accomplished by other means. However, we do so with extreme respect, caution, and reverence for the unique sensitivity and potency of the psoas.

Benefits of psoas work

Many practitioners and clients find benefits from careful psoas work, for a wide variety of reasons (25). Each manual therapy system that includes the psoas in its repertory has its own rationales for doing so. For example, Ida Rolf (the originator of Rolfing Structural Integration) placed special importance on the psoas' role in her work. "A balanced body lengthens," she said. "There is no shortening. If the 'psoas' muscle is where it belongs, the body lengthens in all movement." Her direct techniques often encouraged the psoas to "fall back" within the abdomen (26).

In our Advanced Myofascial Techniques trainings, we work with the psoas as one of many possible avenues for furthering our two primary therapeutic goals, which are:

1. more options for movement, and
2. proprioceptive refinement (27).

In particular, we have observed that careful, direct work with the psoas produces beneficial effects such as:

• immediate and lasting improvements in certain clients' back or sacroiliac pain (both acute and chronic);

• the already-mentioned improvements in nerve entrapment pain in the sciatic, femoral, obturator, genitofemoral distribution areas; and

• client reports of increased awareness and proprioceptive (felt) sense of length, ease, mobility, balance, or continuity through the midsection of the body in standing, walking, and running.

The Psoas Technique, then, is particularly indicated in cases of back pain, nerve pain such as axial sciatica, as well as lumbar, pelvic, or hip joint mobility restrictions. And because of its unique role as a connector of the upper and lower body, as well as its high sensitivity and proprioceptive function, we often use the Psoas Technique in the closing, integrative stages of a session or series. At this stage, the goals have shifted from mobilizing, lengthening, and differentiating specific structures, to awakening proprioceptive awareness of large (broad) relationships in the body, as well as calming, balancing, and completing the hands-on work.

The Psoas Technique (Supine)

Starting with your client supine, ask her to raise her knees (Figure 5.5). This slackens the myofascial layers of the abdominal wall, which helps to make this technique more comfortable and less invasive. We typically don't put a bolster under the knees, as their active involvement in stabilizing the legs helps increase the desired proprioception, and, we will be asking for active movements that a bolster would obstruct.

As you prepare to touch your client, make sure your approach and mindset are soft, sensitive, and unhurried. In Chapter 4, *The Mesentery and the Abdomen*, we described the kind of touch needed for working in the abdomen as similar to touching a soap bubble without bursting it. You'll use the same touch for working with the psoas. The soft visceral and peritoneal tissues of the abdomen are not like the denser myofascial

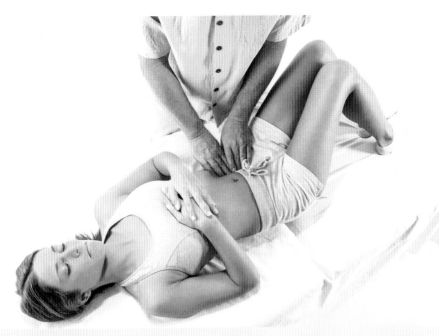

Figure 5.5

The Psoas Technique (supine). Use a patient, delicate touch to gently sink into the client's abdomen. Since one of our primary aims is refined proprioception, the pressure should be very light and sensitive.

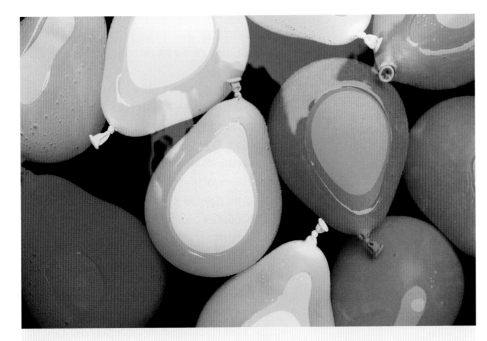

Figure 5.6

The type of touch needed to sensitively and safely work with the psoas in a supine position is akin to feeling in a tub filled with water balloons (the viscera) for a single balloon (the psoas) at the bottom.

tissues of the limbs or spine, and need a different pace, pressure, and presence.

Begin at about the midpoint between the umbilicus and your client's side. Use a delicate, sensing touch, never pushing or pressing. Gently, using the rhythm of your client's breath, allow this soft touch to sink into your client's abdomen. Imagine gently sinking into a tub of water balloons (Figure 5.6), patiently making your way to the bottom as the slippery, delicate balloons (the viscera) slide out of the way. Slowly sink posteromedially—towards the back, and slightly towards the center of the body.

The safest approach is to stay at or below the level of the umbilicus. Above this level, the kidneys and their vasculature lie close to the psoas, and although our touch remains so soft and sensitive that any damage or bruising is unlikely, it's a good practice to stay below (caudal to) the umbilicus, at least until you are very experienced with the kind of patient, listening touch needed in the abdomen.

Stay in close verbal communication with your client, checking in about comfort level, pace, etc. Encourage easy diaphragmatic breathing. Your client's exhalation will draw your hands deeper into the abdominal space. At some point, usually after at least five to ten of these slow, relaxed breaths, you'll stop sinking, and find yourself resting against the slightly firmer posterior abdominal wall. Ask your client to make a very small movement of her leg, lifting the knee towards the ceiling. This will allow you and your client to feel the slight contraction of the psoas. Adjust your position if needed, and repeat, until the contraction of the psoas is clear to you both. Although this area is very sensitive, at no time should the work be painful or unpleasant.

As long as the work is comfortable for your client, you can invite different slow but active movements in order to help your client feel the psoas/leg connection in various ways. Try

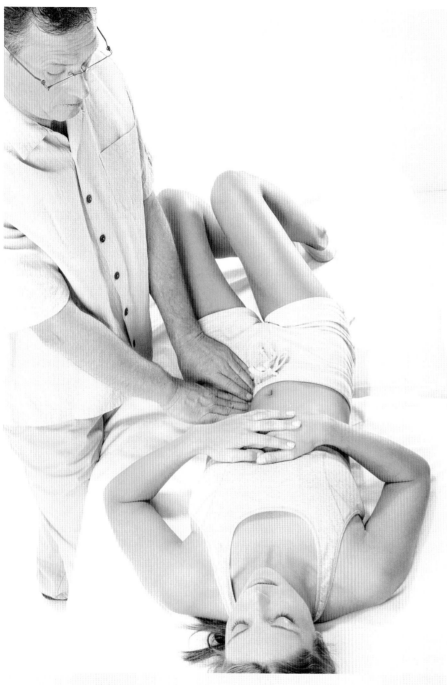

Figure 5.7

After gradually sinking to the level of the psoas, use slow, active hip flexion or side-to-side motion of the raised knees to locate and indicate the psoas' function to your client.

slowly dropping the knees from side-to-side (Figure 5.7), or sliding the leg out along the table. Direct your client to slow down even more, and ease off on your touch if you find movements that are difficult for your client, or particularly sensitive. Once you've both clearly felt the psoas' participation in these various motions, withdraw your touch just as slowly and deliberately as you began. Repeat on the other side.

Psoas Technique (Lateral)

The psoas can also be accessed comfortably with your client in a lateral position (Figure 5.8). This side-lying approach is especially useful when supine work might be difficult or uncomfortable, such as with clients who have a large abdomen.

Key points: Psoas Techniques (Supine and Lateral)

Indications include:
- Low back; sacroiliac joint pain.
- Pain related to lumbar nerve root entrapment, such as femoral nerve pain or axial sciatica.
- Lumbar, pelvic, or hip mobility restrictions.

Purpose
- Increase clients' proprioceptive awareness of psoas function and spine/leg relationship.
- Upper/lower body integration after direct work.

Instructions
1. Sink gently, slowly, and with great sensitivity into the abdominal space. Wait for the viscera to move out of the way. Check in about level, pace, comfort.
2. Once abdomen has softened, ask for active but slow client movement.

Movements
- Gentle hip flexion.
- Drop knees side-to-side (supine) or abduct/adduct upper leg (side-lying).
- Slowly side leg out along the table (hip extension).

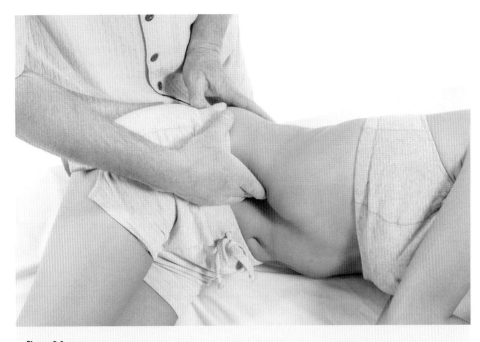

Figure 5.8

The Psoas Technique (Lateral) is useful when a supine version is uncomfortable or difficult. Use the same gentle, soft touch as in the supine variation. Because gravity does not assist with your slow sinking into the abdomen, gentle posterior pressure is necessary to sink, making sensitivity even more important.

Position yourself comfortably behind your client. With the same patient, sensitive, non-pushing touch we used in the supine version, slowly sink backwards. Although the touch is gentle, a bit more effort on the practitioner's part is typically required than in the supine version, since gravity is not an aid in this case. The practitioner's challenge is to remain just as sensitive, slow, and yielding, even when using the small amount of effort required.

As with the supine version, invite the client to initiate gentle active hip flexion (Figure 5.9), as well as hip abduction and adduction, in order to locate, differentiate, and increase awareness of the psoas' actions.

Summary

In contrast to other ways of working with the psoas, the shared goal of these gentle techniques is refined proprioception. This occurs naturally when the sensations of psoas work are gradual and mild enough to be not only tolerated, but actively explored by the client. This enhanced proprioceptive awareness of the psoas is in itself therapeutic and seems to help relieve many conditions, including back pain and other issues. The novel sensations that these techniques evoke are themselves the point of the work, and the gentle intensity of experience means there is often something deeply satisfying about receiving skillful psoas work.

References

[1] Koch, L. (2012) in Tom Myers & Liz Koch, *A Psoas Conversation Part I.* http://www.coreawareness.com/podcasts/apsoasconversation/. [Accessed December 2015]

[2] Platzer, W. (2006) *Thieme Atlas of Anatomy.* Thieme. p. 422–423.

[3] Koch, L. (2012) The psoas is NOT a hip flexor. *Pilates Digest.* http://www.pilatesdigest.com/the-psoas-is-not-a-hip-flexor/. [Accessed December 2015]

[4] Skyrme, A. et al. (1999) Psoas major and its controversial rotational action. *Clinical Anatomy* 12(4). p. 264–265.

[5] Schleip, R. (November 1998) Lecture Notes on Psoas & Adductors. Rolf Institute: *Rolf Lines.*

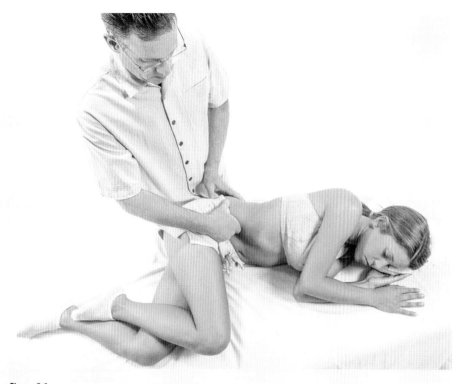

Figure 5.9

As in the supine version, invite gentle, slow, active hip flexion to increase proprioceptive differentiation in The Psoas Technique (Lateral).

[6] Bogduk, N. (1997) *Clinical Anatomy of the Lumbar Spine and Sacrum.* Edinburgh: Churchill Livingstone. p. 102.

[7] Hamill, J. and Knutzen, K.M. (2003) *Biomechanical Basis of Human Movement.* 2nd ed. Baltimore: Lippincott Williams & Wilkins.

[8] Rolf, I.P. (1989) *Rolfing.* Healing Arts Press.

[9] Copaver K. et al. (2012) The effects of psoas major and lumbar lordosis on hip flexion and sprint performance. *Research Quarterly for Exercise and Sport.* 83(2). p. 160–167.

[10] Denmark, D.P. The psoas is involved in most back pain. http://www.bowen.asn.au/bowen-therapy/articles/psoas-muscle-and-back-pain/. [Accessed December 2015]

[11] Ingraham, P. (2015) Psoas, so what? https://www.painscience.com/articles/iliopsoas.php. [Accessed December 2015]

[12] Ingraham, P. (2015) ibid.

[13] Koch, L. (March 2010) The primordial psoas and the Chakra system. *Positive Health.* 168.

[14] Rolf, I.P. (1989) ibid.

[15] Koch, L. (2012) Ibid.

[16] Meakins, A. (March 26, 2014) Psoas... please release me, let me go! *The Sports Physio.* https://thesportsphysio.wordpress.com/2014/03/26/please-release-me-let-me-go/. [Accessed December 2015]

[17] Meakins, A. (2014) ibid.

[18] Hugo, A. et al. (Nov 1, 1978) Scoliosis. *Clinical Symposia.* 30.

[19] Rassner, L. (2011) Lumbar plexus nerve entrapment syndromes as a cause of groin pain in athletes. *Current Sports Medicine Reports.* 10(2). p. 115–120.

[20] Lo, A. (Jan 2015) The Physio Detective blog, http://physiodetective.com/2015/01/21/serious-warning-if-you-do-any-releases-to-your-psoas-or-abs-you-must-read-this/ [Accessed December 2015]

[21] Reich, P. (1989) *Book of dreams.* Dutton Obelisk.

[22] Lowen, A. (1975) *Bioenergetics.* Penguin/Arkana, reissued 1994.

[23] Hanna, T. (1988). *Somatics: Reawakening the Mind's Control of Movement, Flexibility, and Health.* Da Capo Press.

[24] Berceli, D. (2005) *Trauma Releasing Exercises. Book Surge* 14. p. 16.

[25] Various contributors. Deep Tissue Massage: Any benefit from deep tissue massage on the iliopsoas muscle? https://www.zeel.com/t/deep-tissue-massage/expert-answers/any-benefit-from-deep-tissue-massage-on-the-iliopsoas-muscle. [Accessed December 2015]

[26] Rolf, I.P. (1989) ibid.

[27] Luchau, T. (2015) *Advanced Myofascial Techniques, vol. 1.* Handspring Publications.

Picture credits

Figures 5.1, 5.3, and 5.4 Primal Pictures, used by permission.
Figure: 5.2 Jeff Linn, from the Visible Human Data Project.
Figures 5.5, 5.7, 5.8, and 5.9 Advanced-Trainings.com.
Figure 5.6 Thinkstock.

Study Guide

The Psoas

1 **Which of these is listed as one of the main purposes of Psoas Technique (Supine)?**

a to decrease lumbar lordosis
b to refine proprioception
c to increase hip extension
d to increase hip flexion

2 **What analogy is used to describe the recommended approach to palpating the psoas?**

a stretching a resilient exercise band
b working calmly with a furtive animal
c approaching the spiritual aspect of the psoas with respect
d sinking into a tub of water balloons

3 **In the Psoas Technique, the practitioner's action mostly consists of:**

a cross fiber friction
b static contact
c pin and stretch
d deep compression

4 **In the Psoas Technique, why have the client move the leg?**

a movement increases proprioception, which is in itself therapeutic
b to move the viscera out of the way
c to differentiate axial and appendicular sciatica
d to create friction and break up adhesions

5 **According to the text, what is the psoas' role in upright posture?**

a it pulls the spine upright from a flexed position
b it is a primary cause of idiopathic scoliosis
c it plays a proprioceptive role, not only motor
d it pulls the spine upright from an extended position

For Answer Keys, visit www.Advanced-Trainings.com/v2key/

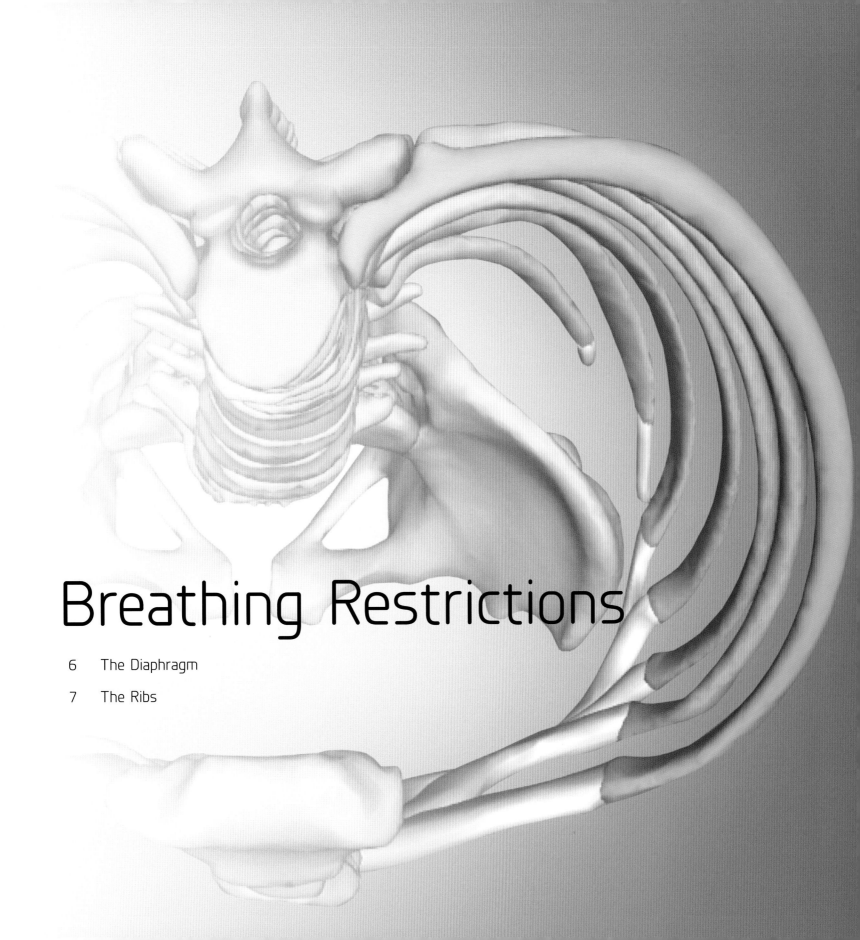

Breathing Restrictions

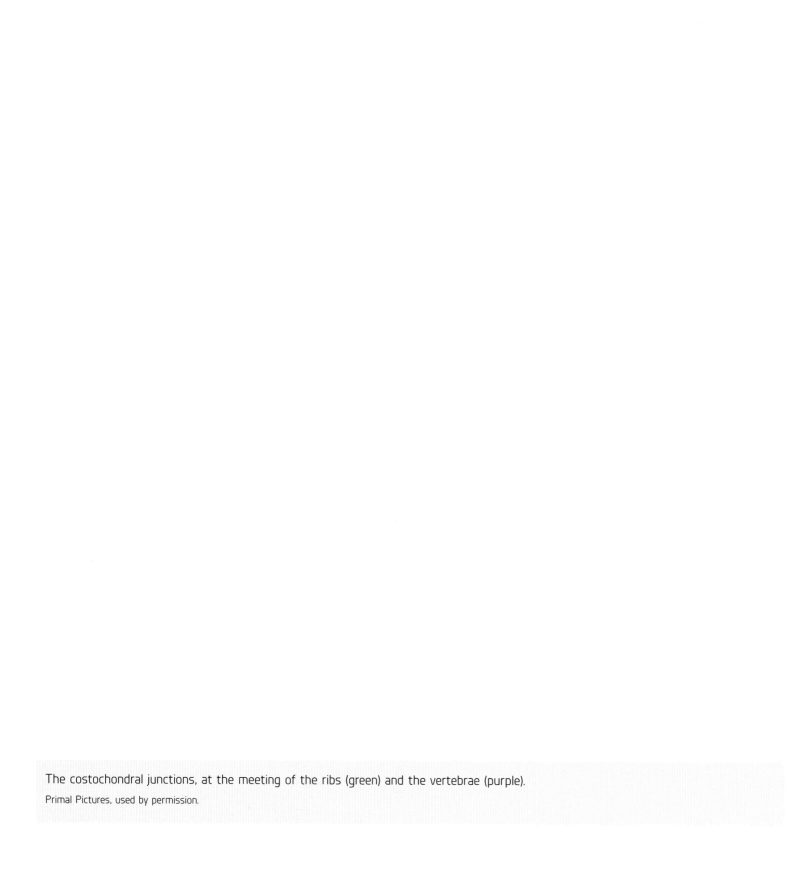

The costochondral junctions, at the meeting of the ribs (green) and the vertebrae (purple).

The Diaphragm

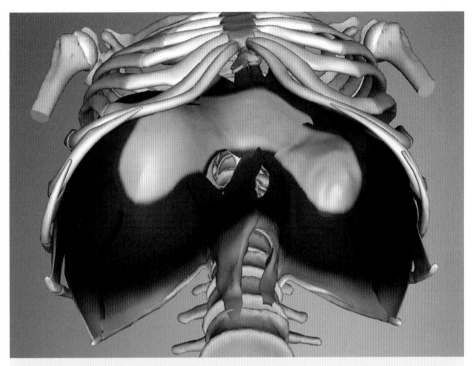

Figure 6.1
The diaphragm attaches all along the lower rim of the bell-like ribcage, as well as to the front of lumbar vertebrae 1–3.

Are you sitting down? Good. Now, take a deep breath. No, I'm not preparing you for bad news—I'm inviting you to explore the movement of your own diaphragm (Figure 6.1).

First, slouch and lean forward a little (Figure 6.2), as if you're furiously typing away on a laptop (maybe writing a chapter in a book). Do you feel how this position can immobilize your diaphragm, crowd your solar plexus, compress your abdomen, and make you breathe more shallowly?

Then, try the opposite: sit up, with your pelvis squarely on your chair, and your feet on the floor. Let your shoulders relax, and breathe into your entire torso. Compare the sensation of this way of breathing to breathing with a crowded midsection. When our diaphragm is free to move, our unrestricted breath flows in and out, rising and falling like gentle ocean waves.

Now, put your hands on your costal arch for your next few breaths. Feel how the ribcage expands and contracts. Imagine the diaphragm, attached all around the lower rim of the bell-like ribcage, moving up and down inside. The diaphragm opens and closes like a slow-motion umbrella (Figures 6.3 and 6.4). As you inhale, the diaphragm contracts, and the umbrella flattens, widens, and moves downward. As you exhale, the diaphragm relaxes, and the umbrella narrows and moves upward into a high dome. Feel this for a few breaths: diaphragm contracting downwards with inhalation; relaxing upwards with your exhalation.

Lastly, compare the front and back of your diaphragm. If you allow your belly to move while you inhale, you'll feel more activity in the front of your diaphragm. Can you do the same with your back? Imagine the posterior, the back part of your diaphragm, expanding in the same way.

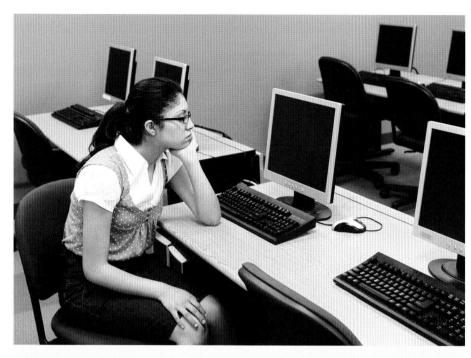

Figure 6.2

Compression and crowding of the anterior diaphragm and the midsection of the thorax.

As Ashtanga yoga teacher Richard Freeman says, "Can you let your kidneys be like miniature wings, expanding and contracting with the breath" (1). Put one hand behind you, if it's hard to feel your breath in this area from the inside out.

Besides its central role in breathing, the diaphragm can contribute to lumbar and low back pain (Figure 6.5), particularly when there is a tendency towards lumbar lordosis. Teaching your clients to find and use the posterior part of the diaphragm when breathing helps refine interoception and proprioception in an area that is often stiff, immobile, and troublesome. As the largest spinal muscle, the diaphragm attaches to the anterior side of the upper three lumbars through its tendinous crura (or "legs"), and along the shafts of the 12th ribs in the small of the back. We addressed working with this region in Chapter 3, *The Iliolumbar Ligament & 12th Rib*. Because the diaphragm acts as an antagonist to the downward pull of the quadratus lumborum on the twelfth ribs, the work with the anterior diaphragm described in this chapter is a perfect complement to the posterior approach in Chapter 3.

Costal Arch/Diaphragm Technique

The respiratory diaphragm's attachments are deep inside the costal arch. Since the diaphragm wraps around the liver, stomach, pancreas, and spleen, its close relationship with these delicate structures makes direct manipulation of the diaphragm inadvisable without specialized in-person training. The liver in particular is vulnerable to bruising or tissue damage; its tissues are so delicate that surgeons removing a lobe of the liver can simply pinch portions of it off with their fingers (2).

Instead of digging under the ribs for the diaphragm, you can safely use the bony edge of

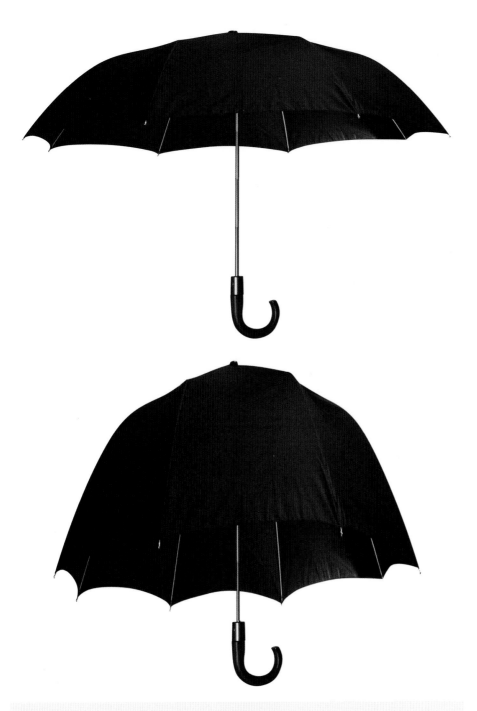

Figures 6.3/6.4

The diaphragm opens and closes with respiration, flattening and widening on inhalation, raising and narrowing with exhalation.

the costal arch to open up the umbrella of the diaphragm in a very effective way, without ever endangering the fragile viscera that the diaphragm surrounds.

Begin the technique by standing at your supine client's side, at the level of his or her hips. Palpate the edge of the costal arch on the opposite side of the body (Figure 6.6). Don't attempt to go under the edge of the costal arch where the diaphragm's actual attachments are. Instead, stay on the bony lower (inferomedial) edge of the costal arch, using a broad, firm, but soft touch to apply gently outward (superolateral) pressure to the very rim of the ribcage. Some people's costal arch is very narrow here; if this is the case, use caution around the sensitive xiphoid process at the end of the sternum.

By reaching across to work the opposite side of your client's body, the angle of your pressure encourages the lower ribs to widen laterally. Wait for your client's breath; on their inhalation, follow the natural widening of the ribcage in order to open and slightly flatten the dome-shaped diaphragm.

Then, when exhalation begins, use your soft but firm touch to hold the costal arch in this widened position, against the pull of the diaphragm from inside. This gently stretches the diaphragm wider as you resist the attempted narrowing of the lower ribcage with exhalation. Feel for the stretch of the diaphragm pulling back at you from inside. By sensitively and softly resisting the diaphragm's narrowing on the exhale, we show the diaphragm what it's like to open a little more with each breath. Repeat this in several places along the costal arch, making sure your touch is comfortable to the client. Any nausea or discomfort are signs that you need to use a different depth or placement. Repeat on the opposite side (Figure 6.7).

Working the diaphragm in this way is an extremely effective way to increase both mobility and proprioception, while being non-invasive and comfortable.

See video of the Coastal Arch/ Diaphragm Technique at www.a-t.tv/sb08

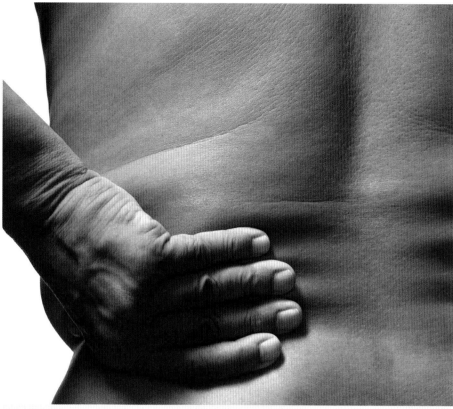

Figure 6.5

The diaphragm can be involved in low back pain through its direct effects on the lumbars, as well as its role as an antagonist to quadratus lumborum at the 12th rib.

Key points: Costal Arch/Diaphragm Technique

Indications include:

- Diminished breath movement in midsection of body.
- Habitually "collapsed" or head-forward postures.
- Morton's neuroma.
- Symptoms related to crowding of the solar plexus and midsection: gastric reflux, heartburn, etc.
- Back, shoulder, jaw, or neck pain.

Purpose

- Refined proprioception related to breath and sitting.
- Increase midsection mobility.

Instructions

With the client supine:

1. Reaching across your client to the opposite side, locate the rim of the costal arch.
2. Apply gentle superolateral (outward) pressure with your client's inhalation, encouraging the ribcage to widen laterally.
3. While your client exhales, hold the costal arch in this slightly widened position, stabilizing against the narrowing of the ribcage.
4. Repeat along length of costal arch.

Cautions

- Do not attempt to work inside the costal arch (in order to avoid damage to delicate viscera).
- Use caution around the sensitive xiphoid process.

Does the diaphragm stabilize the core?

Do we want the diaphragm to relax, or tighten? Doesn't a soft core contribute to back pain? Contraction of the diaphragm does contribute, at least temporarily, to lumbar stability by acting as a lid on the "core" abdominal space. An example of this is the Valsalva maneuver, where forced

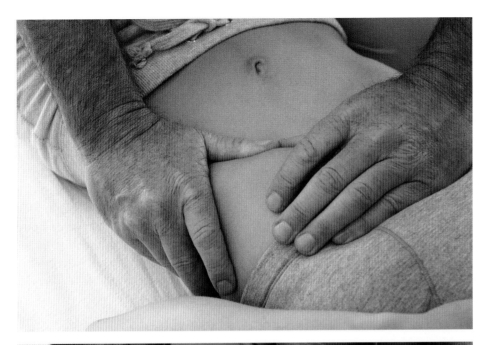

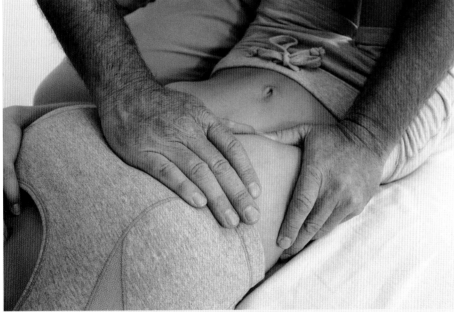

Figures 6.6/6.7

In the Diaphragm/Costal Arch Technique, we avoid endangering the delicate viscera by working solely with the bony rim of the costal arch, rather than trying to touch the diaphragm's attachments inside the ribcage. Work across the body, following the costal arch as it widens inhalation, then maintaining that width with gentle pressure as exhaling stretches the diaphragm.

exhalation is pressed against a closed airway. This technique is used (both intentionally and unintentionally) by weightlifters to add additional support during a heavy lift by increasing intra-abdominal pressure, which temporarily stiffens the lumbar segment. Electromyographic studies show the diaphragm also contracts to support shoulder movements (3) and its central position in the body, it likely acts as a stabilizer in many other motions as well.

However, since we can't hold our breath all the time, some writers argue that asking the diaphragm to constantly act as a core stabilizer inhibits the responsiveness and flexibility needed in its role as a continually expanding and contracting structure (4). A diaphragm that lacks movement flexibility is not an asset—think of hiccups, or even worse, the immobility of having the wind knocked out of you. Both are examples of the diaphragm in a spasm of contraction. By contrast, a flexible, responsive diaphragm is what allows the breath to move freely and fully. Increased mobility and proprioception (our twin goals of the Advanced Myofascial Techniques approach) allow the diaphragm to more fully respond to the changing demands placed on it: stability and strength at those moments when they are needed, with flexibility and adaptability as its resting state.

Other diaphragms

The structure we have been discussing is more accurately called the respiratory diaphragm, as it is only one of the diaphragms of the body. The word diaphragm comes to us directly from the ancient Greek διάφραγμα or "partition." Some of the other anatomical structures that are conventionally considered to be diaphragms include the urogenital diaphragm (between the pelvic rami) and the pelvic diaphragm (or pelvic floor) which supports the pelvic organs, and forms the lower

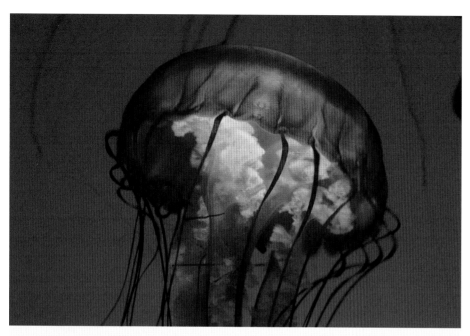

Figure 6.8

The movement of the diaphragm in breathing can be much like the undulating opening and closing of a jellyfish.

end of the abdominal space bounded by the respiratory diaphragm at its upper end.

Rolfing structural integration (and osteopathic traditions) refer to several other horizontal myofascial structures as diaphragms. The soles of the feet, the menisci, the perineum, the thoracic outlet, the roof of the mouth, and the cranial tentorium are all considered to have diaphragm-like qualities or motion potential. In structural integration, the functional and anatomical interrelationships of these structures are thought to play a part in balanced alignment and whole-body integration (5), for example, imagine the soles of your feet "breathing" like your respiratory diaphragm does, opening and closing to receive the weight transfer of each step.

Summary

The respiratory diaphragm plays many roles in the body—breathing, containing, stabilizing, supporting the low back, and more. It cycles through expansion and contraction in all dimensions, with every breath. Helping our clients increase their felt sense of diaphragmatic spaciousness, freedom, and openness will be much appreciated, and will help support your mobility and proprioception goals in other parts of the body.

We began by paying attention to the movements of our own diaphragm, contrasting what it does when we are slumped with the felt sense of sitting more upright. Return to your own diaphragm now, feeling the slow, tidal movements of the gentle expansion and contraction of each breath. When it's free, the diaphragm moves much like a jellyfish does—floating in its fluid environment, changing its shape within its 360 degrees of movement possibility (Figure 6.8). This rhythmic opening and closing of the diaphragm causes the organs around it to undulate and drift with the breath, like other nearby jellyfish moving with the swell. Why not take some time now to just enjoy the waves?

References

[1] Freeman, R. (1992) *Personal communication*.

[2] Poon, T.P. (2007). Current techniques of liver transection. *HPB: The Official Journal of the International Hepato Pancreato Biliary Association (Oxford)*. 9(3). p. 166–173.

[3] Richardson, C. et al. (1999) *Therapeutic Exercise for Spinal Segmental Stabilization in Low Back Pain*. Edinburgh: Churchill Livingstone.

[4] Newton, A., (2004) Writing about Hubert Goddard in *Core Stabilization, Core Coordination*. http://www.alinenewton.com/pdf-articles/core.htm. [Accessed December 2015.]

[5] ibid.

Picture credits

Figures 6.1, 6.3, 6.4, and 6.5 Thinkstock.

Figure 6.2 Primal Pictures, used by permission.

Figures 6.6 and 6.7 Advanced-Trainings.com.

Study Guide

The Diaphragm

1 **With inhalation, the respiratory diaphragm:**

a contracts, flattens, widens, moves upward
b contracts, flattens, widens, moves downward
c relaxes, flattens, widens, moves downward
d relaxes, flattens, narrows, moves upward

2 **The text says that the respiratory diaphragm is the largest muscle of the:**

a abdomen
b thorax
c back
d body

3 **What is the interaction between the quadratus lumborum and the respiratory diaphragm?**

a indirect: they do not share a direct attachment
b antagonistic: the quadratus lumborum pulls up on the 12th rib, while the diaphragm pulls down
c agonistic: the diaphragm pulls up on the 12th rib and the quadratus lumborum assists
d antagonistic: the diaphragm pulls up on the 12th rib, while the quadratus lumborum pulls down

4 **The purpose of the Costal Arch/Diaphragm Technique is:**

a to increase stability during heavy lifting by building core stability
b to decrease frequency and severity of hiccups, side-stitches, and spasms
c to increase midsection mobility and proprioception
d to differentiate the fascia of the diaphragmatic perimysium from the pleural fascia

5 **In the Costal Arch/Diaphragm Technique, the practitioner creates a gentle stretch by:**

a resisting the movement of the ribs on the inhale
b resisting the movement of the ribs on the exhale
c assisting the movement of the ribs on the exhale
d assisting the movement of the diaphragm on the inhale

For Answer Keys, visit www.Advanced-Trainings.com/v2key/

The Ribs

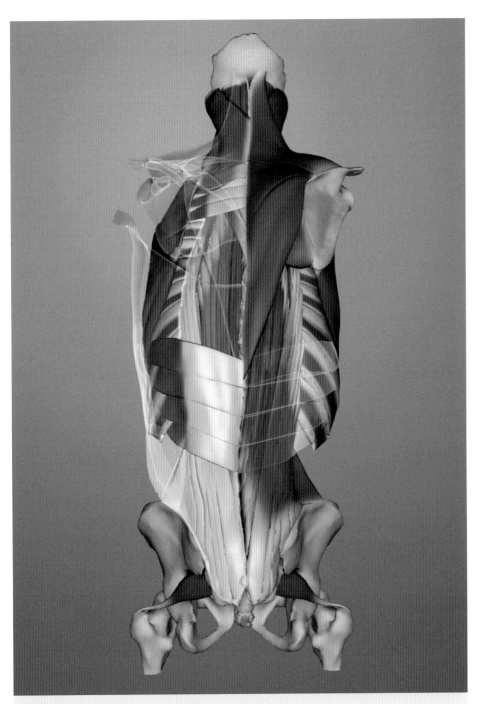

Figure 7.1

The ribs lie deep to many of the shoulder girdle and back's soft tissue structures. Prepare for rib work by addressing these first. The erector group's iliocostalis (yellow) and longissimus thoracis (violet) directly attach to the ribs, as does their surrounding thoracolumbar fascia (green).

The ribs

Take a breath. How much did your ribcage move, and where? Take another breath, this time without moving your ribs as much. Did you notice the unpleasant, hard-to-breathe sensation? That's what restricted rib motion feels like, whether the restrictions are from connective tissue constriction, pain, posture, or habit.

Breath efficacy affects a wide range of functions, from metabolic processes, to our energy level, alertness, and mood (1). Since we take approximately 24,000 breaths in a day, even small changes in our respiratory efficiency will have cumulative and far-reaching body-mind effects. Fortunately, this multiplying effect works both ways: not only can breath restrictions make us feel bad, but even small, incremental improvements in rib freedom can improve our well-being on many levels.

Restricted rib motion can arise from the usual things that cause us to lose mobility: stress, habitual posture and stance, inactivity, disease, pain, fear, and injury. The ribs serve as a protective cage around our most vital organs, shielding our heart, lungs, and liver. But they must also be flexible enough to allow for another vital function: breath.

No matter what the cause, skilled hands-on work can be an effective way to help re-establish lost motion and adaptability. But, before using the techniques in this chapter, we'll begin our work with the back.

Erector Technique

Your work with rib restrictions will be more effective if you take time to release the larger, more superficial structures around the ribcage first, particularly the erector spinae group. Within the erector spinae group, (Figure 7.1),

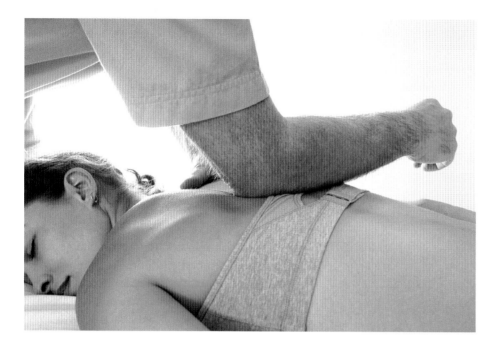

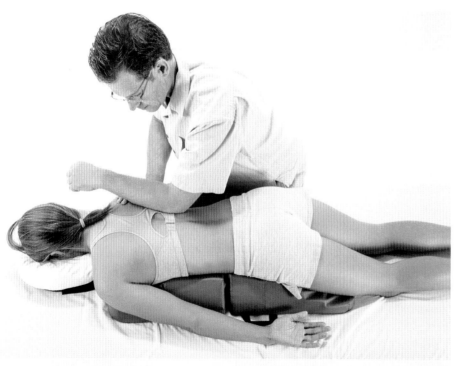

Figures 7.2/7.3

Use the flat portion of your forearm to differentiate the fascia around and within the iliocostalis group, the most lateral of the erector spinae.

the iliocostalis, the longissimus thoracis, and their surrounding thoracolumbar fascia connect ribs to other structures, and will restrict breath mobility when tight (both fascial stiffness and high muscle tone are common here). You will also find it easier to assess the movement of the ribs themselves in the subsequent techniques if you release the erector spinae group first. Use the Erector Technique (Chapter 1) or similar to prepare the outer layers of back myofascia before attempting the deeper work here.

The forearm tool is an effective way to work with the erectors. Without using oil or lubricant (which would eliminate the slight friction necessary to differentiate individual layers), use your forearm to apply a bit of caudal (downward) pressure on the erectors (Figure 7.2), feeling for their lateral edge. At first, feel for variations in tissue density, rather than attempting to release or change the tissue. Keep your other, non-working hand on your client, close to your forearm. This will stabilize your body position, and give you a bigger "footprint" in your client's awareness, which will help him or her relax into your touch. Allow the slow release of the tissue to set the pace for your gradual gliding movement down the back. Begin with moderate pressure, in order to prepare and warm up the superficial layers. Once they've released, on your successive passes feel deeper into the back's myofascia, working slowly, layer by layer. Surrounding the erector group is the highly sensitive thoracolumbar fascia; it, among other structures, has been implicated in otherwise unexplained back pain (Chapter 1) (10). You might ask your client to let the breath gently expand under your touch. This will help to release from the inside the same places you're working from the outside.

Locally dense areas can sometimes be more directly addressed by working in a cephalad (upward) direction (Figure 7.3). Work the entire length of the erectors, but be extra-sensitive over the lower floating ribs and the lumbars.

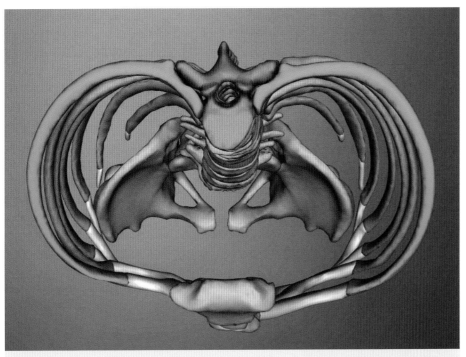

Figure 7.4
The oblique angle of the costovertebral joints means the ribs (green) are anterolateral to the transverse processes of the vertebrae (purple).

Costovertebral Joint Technique

One of the most commonly overlooked places where ribs lose mobility is at the costovertebral joints, where the ribs articulate with the spine. Deep to the erectors, the area around these key joints is filled with ligaments and small muscles, which when shortened or hard, can bind the ribs and vertebrae together into an immobile mass. Free costovertebral joints allow the ribs to change their angle in relation to the spine, lifting with inhalation, and dropping with exhalation. Since the costovertebral joints are obliquely arranged, with the rib lying anterolateral to the transverse processes of the vertebrae (Figure 7.4), these joints also allow a small amount of anterior rib movement as well. This anterior movement is an indicator of freedom at this joint.

Assess this anterior mobility after you've worked the erectors with the previous technique. With your client prone, use what manual therapy teacher Art Riggs calls the "piano key" method

(3): using either your fingers, thumbs, palm, or forearm (as in the Erector Technique, Figure 7.2), check each rib's anterior mobility in turn. Each rib can be palpated just lateral to the muscle mass of the erectors, or on the upper ribs, just medial to the scapula. A variation is to reach under your supine client, and with your fingertips, lift each rib from underneath.

Whichever position or assessment method you choose, be sure you're feeling for the bony hardness of the rib itself, and not getting distracted by any remaining tightness in the soft tissues over the ribs or in the laminar groove. Each rib should give slightly when you put anterior pressure on it. An unyielding rib or particular tenderness with the "piano key" method test reveals an issue with that rib's costovertebral joints (Figure 7.4). Test all ribs, using caution and very little pressure on the lowest two pairs of floating ribs.

Once you've identified which costovertebral joints are restricted, position your client on his or her side, with the restricted joint on the upper side (for example, for right-side restrictions, your client would lie on her left side). Curl your client into a tight fetal position, with hips and spine in tight flexion, knees to the chest, and chin tucked. This position will give you a head start by creating a bit more space between adjacent vertebral transverse processes, opening them away from the neck of the restricted rib.

Using the flat section of your ulna just distal to your elbow, apply pressure (in an anterior and slightly medial direction, Figure 7.5) to the back (posterior angle) of the restricted ribs (Figure 7.6). Usually it is most effective to approach at a low angle, almost parallel to the table. Adjust the direction of your pressure until you feel the rib itself; then, lean into it. Make sure your client is comfortable, and wait for a release. You can invite your client to breathe

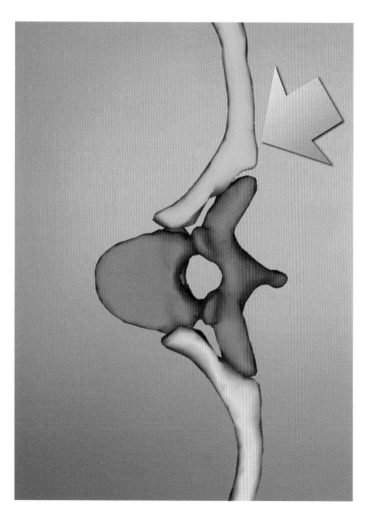

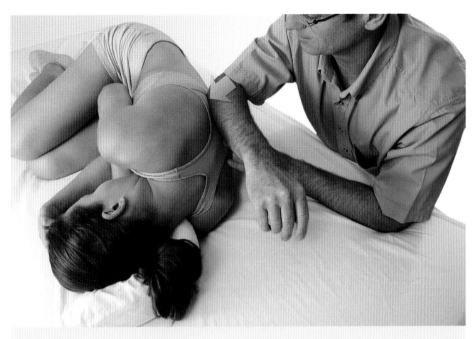

Figures 7.5/7.6

Applying gentle, steady anteromedial pressure (arrow) to assess and encourage rib mobility in the Costovertebral Joint Technique. Note flexed client position.

into his or her back, which will fill the area you're working with and encourage the spine to move slightly posteriorly. You can monitor this slight posterior motion of the spine with your non-working hand. The key here is patience; stay comfortable in your own body so that you can sustain the pressure for several breaths, giving the ligaments around the joints time to respond. You'll feel the rib become subtly but tangibly mobile if you wait long enough.

When you've released the restrictions on one side, turn your client over and work the restrictions on his or her other side, so that you're working the upper side again. Or, before your client turns over, check another dimension of that side's rib mobility with the Bucket Handle Technique—also called the Intercostal Space Technique.

Key points: Costovertebral Joint Technique

Indications include:
- Rib, shoulder, or thoracic back pain.
- Local rib or global ribcage immobility.

Purpose
- Mobilize rib restrictions at the costovertebral joints.

Instructions

With client prone or supine, assess each rib's anterior mobility and sensitivity to pain (the "piano key" assessment):

1. Reposition client into a side-lying, tightly flexed position.
2. Use forearm to apply static, patient pressure in an anterior and slightly medial direction to the posterior angle of any restricted ribs.
3. Adjust your angle, feeling for maximum effect; lean, cue breath, and wait for rib to subtly "drift" or yield anteriorly.

Movements
- Focused, gentle breath into the back.

See video of the Intercostal Space Technique at www.a-t.tv/sb05

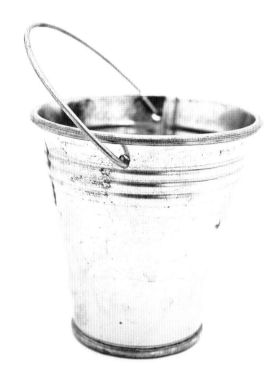

Figure 7.7

The ribs articulate at their posterior and anterior ends, so ribcage expansion causes individual ribs to rise on inhalation, much like a bucket handle pivots on its fastened ends.

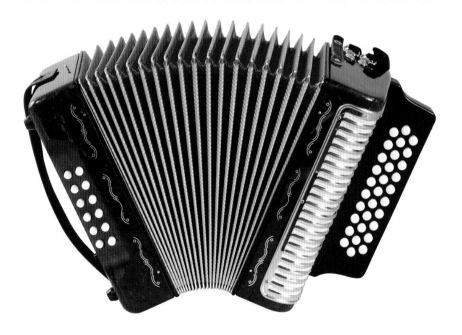

Intercostal Space Technique

Once you've addressed restrictions at the costovertebral joints, you can proceed around the rib's shaft to check for the ribs' cranial/caudal motion. Since the ribs articulate at their posterior and anterior ends, ribcage expansion causes their most lateral part to rise on inhalation, much like a bucket handle pivots on its fastened ends when lifted (Figure 7.7). This motion depends on the mobility not only of the costovertebral joints, but on the ability of the intercostal structures to lengthen and allow separation between the ribs (4).

To check the ribs' ability to separate, position yourself behind your side-lying client, facing the foot of the table. Your client should no longer be in the tight fetal position of the Costovertebral Joint Technique, but lying with the spine straight, that is, neither flexed nor extended. Use a broad open hand to check for expansion between the ribs as you direct your client to take a full breath. When the ribs are free, you'll feel each intercostal space expand on inhalation, much like the pleats of an accordion expand (Figure 7.8). Note any rib spaces that expand less than others. Most of us have restrictions here; for example, on women, the spaces at the level of a bra-strap can become bound together by restricted fascia, and move together as a group, instead of as individual bones.

To address any restricted intercostal spaces you find, use the base of your forefinger at the edge of your hand to apply gentle caudal (inferior) pressure to the upper edge of the rib, below the restricted intercostal space (Figure 7.9). For example, if the intercostal space between ribs four and five is restricted, apply inferior pressure to the upper edge of rib five, thus encouraging the restricted space above rib five to opening with direct but gentle pressure.

In fact, your pressure itself will not open the space, as much as your client's breath will. Once your hands are in position, ask your client to "inhale above this place," as you resist the tendency of the lower rib to lift with inspiration. It may take your client a few attempts to discover how to lift the ribs above your stabilizing hands. Patiently coach your client to be specific with their in-breath, "inhaling from here up." This motion will actively separate the ribs, and open restricted intercostal spaces.

Depending on your client's tendency towards exhalation- or inhalation-fixation, sometimes it is more effective to reverse the technique, stabilizing a rib superiorly while the client actively exhales below that level (Figure 7.10). In this version, the contraction of the abdomen and internal intercostals in forcible exhalation pulls the ribs downward. When combined with your gentle upward pressure on the rib just above the restricted space, you can use the exhalation (instead of an inhalation) to open a restricted intercostal space (Figure 7.11). If one variation does not seem particularly effective with your client's intercostal restrictions, try the opposite approach. The release will be clear to both you and your client when you get it right.

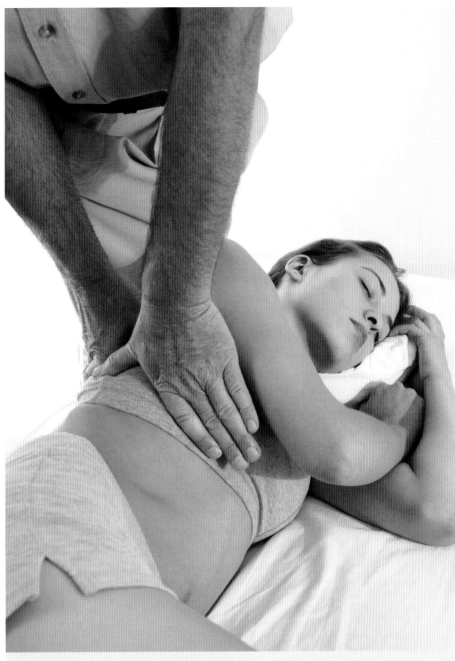

Figures 7.8/7.9
Stabilizing a rib against the lift of active inhalation in the Intercostal Space Technique allows the intercostal spaces to open like the pleats of an accordion.

Key points: Intercostal Space Technique

Indications include:
- Ribcage, breath, or thoracic sidebending restrictions.
- Scoliosis.

Purpose
- Increase ribs' "bucket handle" mobility.

Instructions and Movement
1. Feel or watch for expansion and contraction of each intercostal space with full breathing.
2. Use edge of hand to caudally stabilize the rib below restricted space.
3. Cue client to inhale "above this place" to lift ribs, expanding the intercostal space.
4. Alternatively, stabilize the rib above the restricted space, and ask for exhalation "below this place" to drop ribs and expand the intercostal space.

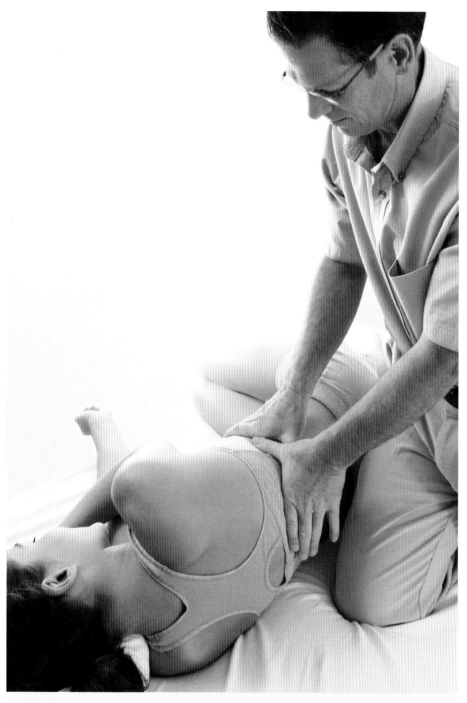

Figure 7.10

The Intercostal Space Technique, reversed: stabilizing a rib against the downward pull of exaggerated exhalation to open the intercostal space below the stabilized rib.

Rib pain considerations

The techniques described here are effective in reducing many kinds of rib pain, including mild rib displacements or fixations. It is important to keep in mind that in addition to soft tissue or articular restrictions, rib pain can accompany other issues, including these:

- Bruised, cracked, or fractured ribs; or costochondritis (inflammation of the sternal cartilage, usually painful but benign) often respond best to rest and the passage of time. Once healed, these can leave behind tissue and movement restrictions that these techniques can help relieve.
- Pleurisy (inflamed linings of the lung cavity) should be considered when breathing is painful. Referral to a physician is indicated when pleurisy is suspected.
- Cardiac issues can also cause chest pain. In the most cautious approach, unexplained chest pain should be considered an emergency until cardiac issues can be ruled out.
- Osteoporosis (a bone disease that increases the risk of fracture) initially has few signs or symptoms unless a fracture has already occurred, and is difficult to detect without screening (5). Both men and women can be affected. Bone density screening is recommended when three or more of these risk factors are present: being over age 65, Caucasian or Asian, female, low body weight, or a family history of osteoporosis. Play it safe and avoid excessive pressure on the ribs or spine when you suspect any risk of osteoporosis.

By assessing and releasing restrictions to the ribs' mobility at their articulations and intercostal spaces, we increase our effectiveness and the contribution we make towards our clients' overall well-being.

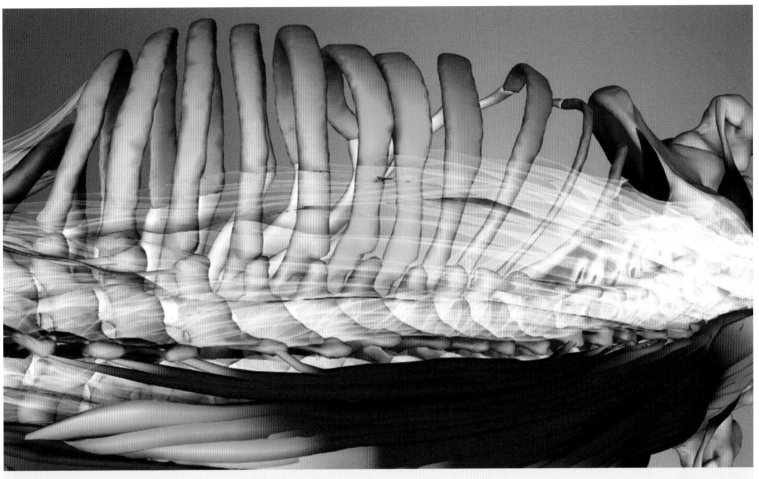

Figure 7.11

A narrower intercostal space. The erector group is transparent on the top (client's right) side.

References

[1] Two studies on the link between breathing and depression: 1) Brown, R.P. et al. (2005) Sudarshan Kriya yogic breathing in the treatment of stress, anxiety, and depression: Part I—Neurophysiologic model. *Journal of Alternative and Complementary Medicine.* 11(1). p. 189–201. 2) Tweeddale, P.M., Rowbottom, I., and McHardy, G.J. (1994) Breathing retraining: Effect on anxiety and depression scores in behavioural breathlessness. *Journal of Psychosomatic Research.* 38(1). p. 11–21.

[2] Langevin, H.M. et al. (2011) Reduced thoracolumbar fascia shear strain in human chronic low back pain. *BMC Musculoskeletal Disorders.* 12. p. 203.

[3] Riggs, A. (February 2011) *Personal communication.*

[4] Kapandji, I.A. (2008) *Physiology of the Joints, Vol. III.* New York: Churchill Livingstone. 6th ed. p. 141.

[5] Salvo, S. (2013) *Mosby's Pathology for Massage Therapist.* 3rd ed. Elsevier p. 113.

Picture credits

Figures 7.1, 7.4, 7.5, and 7.11 Primal Pictures, used by permission.
Figures 7.2, 7.3, 7.6, 7.9, and 7.10 Advanced-Trainings.com.
Figures 7.7 and 78 Thinkstock.

Study Guide

The Ribs

1 **Why does the author recommend starting on the erectors of the back?**

a compressing the ribs from behind helps release them from the front
b client will relax faster, making the work more efficient
c tightness and hypertonicity in the erectors will restrict rib mobility
d the ribs are too delicate to work from the front

2 **What client action is suggested in the Erector Technique?**

a breathe into the practitioner's touch, releasing restrictions from the inside
b flex and extend the spine by lifting the head off the table
c slide elbow slowly up and down the table with exhale and inhale
d exhale and hold while the practitioner leans more deeply into the tissue

3 **Freedom at which of these joints will most allow the ribs to lift and drop with the breath?**

a the sternoclavicular joints
b the intervertebral joints
c the scapulocostal joints
d the costovertebral joints

4 **What does the "piano key" method most directly assess?**

a intercostal space openness
b tonicity of the erector group
c posterior mobility of the ribs
d anterior mobility of the ribs

5 **According to the text, why position the client in a tight fetal position for the Costovertebral Joint Technique?**

a the position allows the practitioner to use gravity rather than strength
b the position opens the space between neighboring transverse processes
c the flexed position of the spine is a good counterstretch for prone positions
d the position closes the space between neighboring transverse processes

For Answer Keys, visit www.Advanced-Trainings.com/v2key/

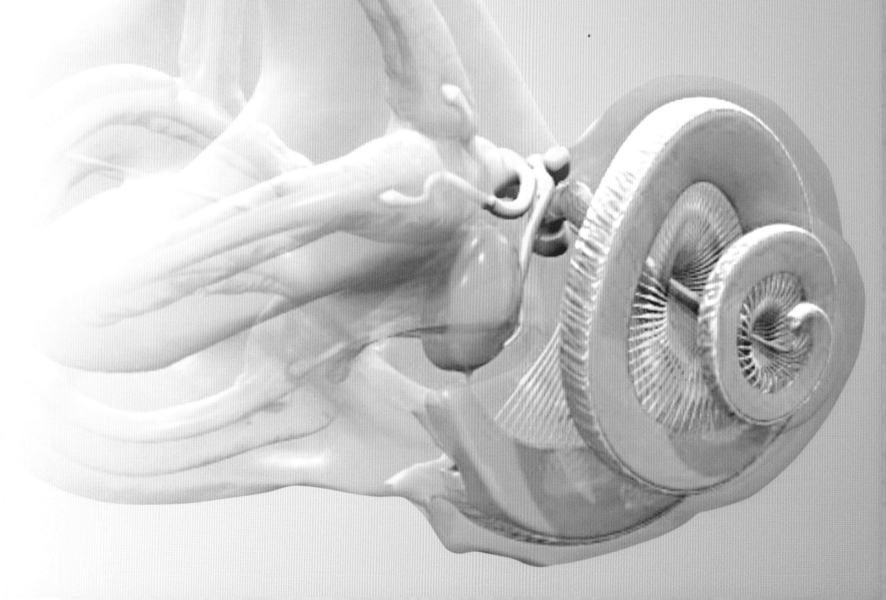

Whiplash

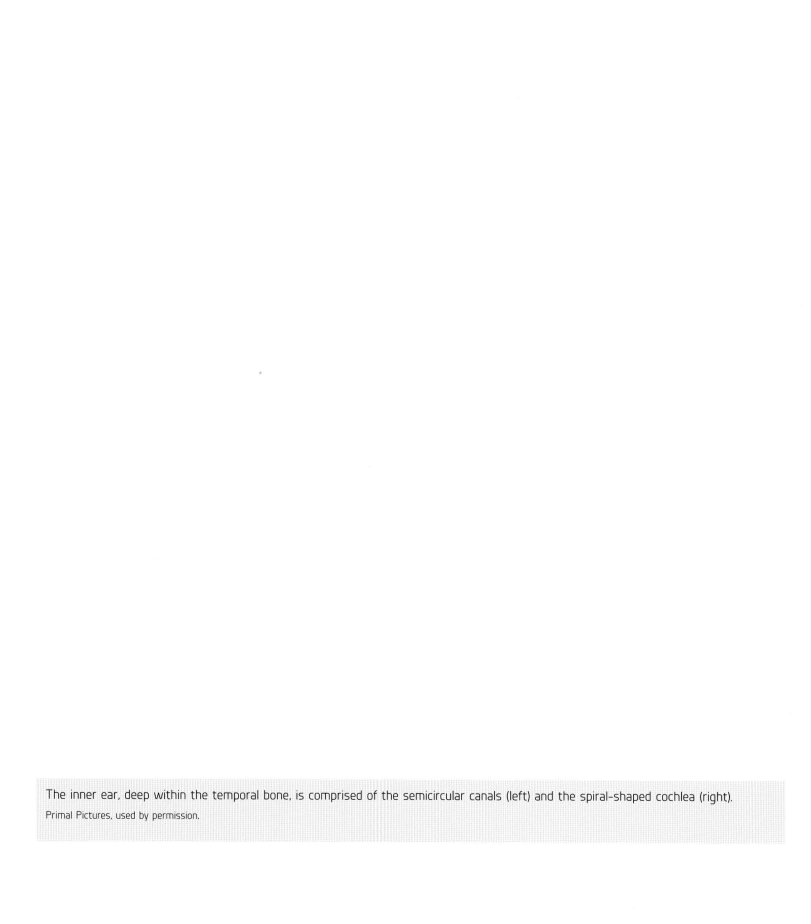

The inner ear, deep within the temporal bone, is comprised of the semicircular canals (left) and the spiral-shaped cochlea (right).

Which way is up? It is such a simple question, but with such large implications. Whenever you are upright, your body orients itself to gravity and to your surroundings, trying to keep your eyes and head level. This sense of "up" provides a point of reference for balance, movement, posture, and position.

An even more important question might be "Which way is down?" Having a stable, trustworthy base of support is one of the body's prerequisites for ease. Imagine trying to stand upright on top of a teetering stepladder—what happens in your body? Do you tighten, stiffen, or clench? This involuntary gripping reaction is triggered, to a greater or lesser degree, whenever your body senses instability or disrupted equilibrium. A neck affected by whiplash, an unstable ankle, or a painful sacroiliac joint are just a few examples of the many conditions that can throw off our body's fundamental sense of stability and orientation. Equilibrium is, of course, a whole-body phenomenon; for the purpose of simplicity, I will focus on the vestibular system in this chapter, which is the single greatest contributor to the body's sense of balance.

Together with the cochlea, which is the sense organ of hearing (Figure 8.2), the vestibular system constitutes the labyrinth of the inner ear (Figure 8.1). Arising from the ectoderm— the same embryonic layer that gives rise to the nervous system, eyes, and skin— the inner ear is the first sense organ to form in the embryo, first appearing at about 22 days of development (1) (Figure 8.3). Interestingly, the inner, middle, and outer ear each arise from different embryonic layers, reflecting their different functions. By six to eight weeks after fertilization, an embryo has developed the inner ear's semicircular canals, making the sensation of movement our earliest sensory experience.

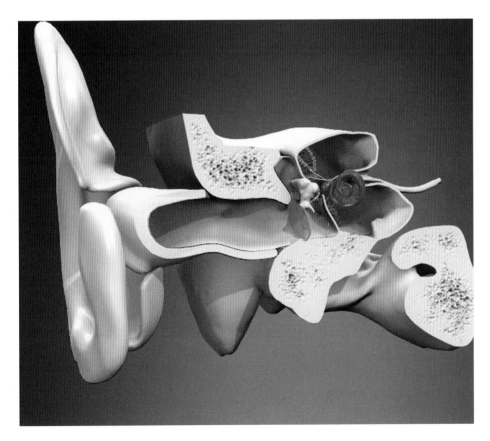

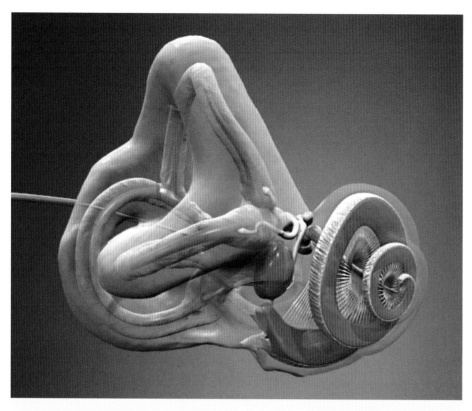

Figures 8.1/8.2

The labyrinth of the inner ear is embedded deep within the skull's temporal bone. It is comprised of the spiraling cochlea, which perceives sound, and the fluid-filled semicircular canals (green, 8.1), which sense movement.

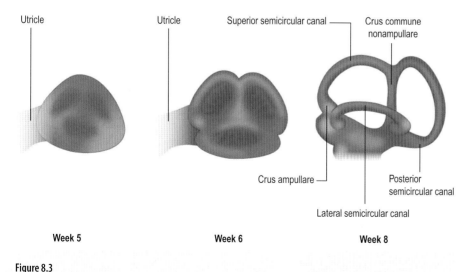

Utricle

Utricle

Superior semicircular canal

Crus commune nonampullare

Crus ampullare

Posterior semicircular canal

Lateral semicircular canal

Week 5   Week 6   Week 8

Figure 8.3

The inner ear is the first sense organ to form in the embryo. The semicircular canals (on the left of Figure 8.2) sense movement, while the spiral-shaped cochlea and its associated nerves (on the right of Figure 8.2) perceive sound.

The vestibular system detects head movement; the central nervous system then uses this information to coordinate body and eye motions. Through its remarkably geometrical arrangement of three interconnected fluid-filled semicircular canals in each ear (Figure 8.4), the vestibular system can detect straight or rotational motion in any of the three ordinal planes. Since we have two ears, the brain can compare left and right vestibular signals, as it does with stereo sound, which helps us distinguish between subtly different experiences, such as differentiating between the force of gravity and the mechanically identical forces of acceleration and deceleration.

The vestibular system detects two types of motion—rotational and linear. Rotational motions of the head (such as turning from side to side, tilting, looking up, or nodding) causes fluid in the semicircular canals to rush by specialized mechanoreceptors called the *ampullary cupulae* (Figure 8.5), which are embedded with sensitive hair-like cells (Figure 8.6). Depending on which way they are bent by the fluid, these hair cells either open or close ion channels in their corresponding nerves, transducing the fluid's motion to a nerve impulse, which is processed in the brain. Linear motions, such as an elevator dropping or an airplane taking off, are detected by other hair cells elsewhere in the inner ear, which sense the inertia of embedded calcium carbonate crystals called *otoliths* (Figure 8.6).

One common form of persistent dizziness or vertigo (benign paroxysmal positional vertigo, or BPPV) is thought to be caused by these otoliths (sometimes known as "ear stones") working free and tumbling to parts of the semicircular canals where they are not usually found. This over-stimulates the hair cells in those areas, and floods the brain's processing centers with unexpected, random signals. This unpleasant condition can often be managed by practicing a series

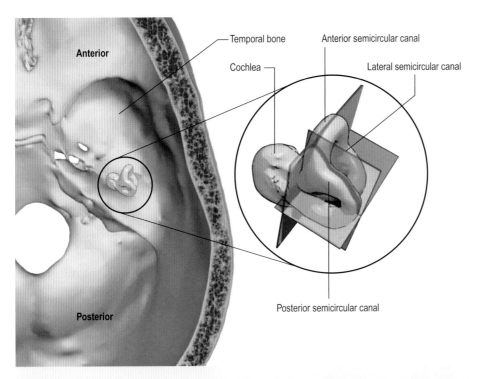

Figure 8.4

The three semicircular canals of each ear are arranged orthogonally, and can sense movement in each of the three dimensions.

of movements, such as Epley's exercises, that tumble the stones back into areas of the canals that do not stimulate vertigo.

Though often performed by a doctor, chiropractor, or physical therapist, clients can learn Epley's maneuvers for self-treatment from any number of sources on the Internet. However, it is important to remember that there are other possible causes of vertigo—some of which require medical care—so persistent, unexplained vertigo is a sufficient reason to refer your client to a physician for evaluation. In any case, if Epley's maneuvers or other movements make the dizziness worse, they should only be used under a trained practitioner's supervision. This said, for vertigo caused by BPPV, Epley's exercises have a very high success rate and are relatively benign (2).

Vertigo is not the only reason we should include the vestibular system in our thinking. Even small amounts of vestibular input can have significant effects in the body. Many studies have linked vestibular stimulation to sympathetic (fight or flight) autonomic nervous system activation and physical reactions such as higher blood pressure, respiratory changes, and increased muscular tension throughout the body (3).

Vestibular disquiet can also trigger body/mind reactions. Moshe Feldenkrais, a prominent body therapy pioneer, postulated that humans begin their process of growth and learning with just one built-in purpose, the "fear of falling" (4). His contemporary and colleague, Ida Rolf, the originator of Rolfing structural integration, is purported to have said, "Ninety-five percent of all neurosis is the fear of falling down." Though both of their statements were probably more hyperbole than substantiated fact, the underlying point is valid: our physical functioning—in this case, the functioning of our vestibular

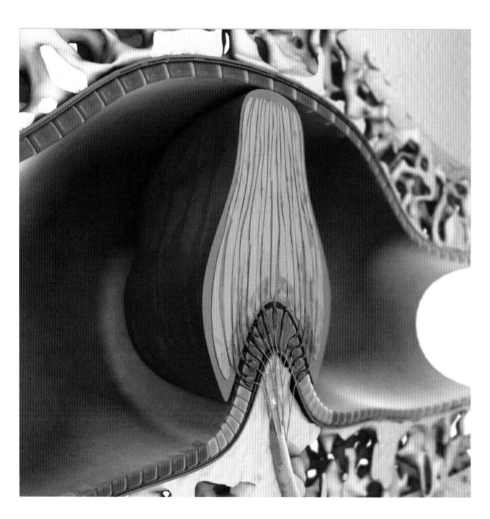

system—strongly influences our psychology, emotions, and inner state.

In hands-on work, we can use this body/mind relationship to our advantage. When disturbed, the vestibular system causes sympathetic fight-or-flight activation, anxiety, tension, and unrest. Change in the opposite direction is possible too: when soothed, supported, and steadied, the vestibular system can trigger a palliative, quieting, relaxing, and calming response instead.

Vestibular Orienting Technique

Due to its power to relax and calm, the Vestibular Orienting Technique is useful in the initial, preparatory phases of a manual therapy session, where it can be an effective way to focus and quiet your client's attention. It is also an effective technique for reducing stress responses. For these reasons, we also use it as a starting point for many instances of "hot" whiplash, unless it triggers guarding or pain (see Chapter 9, *Hot Whiplash*). Additionally, when done with care, this technique can be very effective for reducing vertigo itself, as it is a simple and effective way to assess and reduce vestibular hypersensitivity and disturbance (see the special considerations below).

Begin the technique by slowly lifting your client's head, gently flexing the neck. If your client suffers from vertigo, neck pain, or "hot" whiplash signs (spasm, guarding, or pain), ask him to keep his eyes open, and lift the client's head slowly enough to avoid triggering any dizziness or pain. If the dizziness or pain is acute, you may only be able to lift half an inch; however, in most clients without pain or dizziness, you will be able to slowly take the chin to the chest without triggering discomfort or guarding reactions. Increasing the range of cervical flexion is not the goal; focus instead on sensing your client's comfortable limit; this serves as the starting point of the technique.

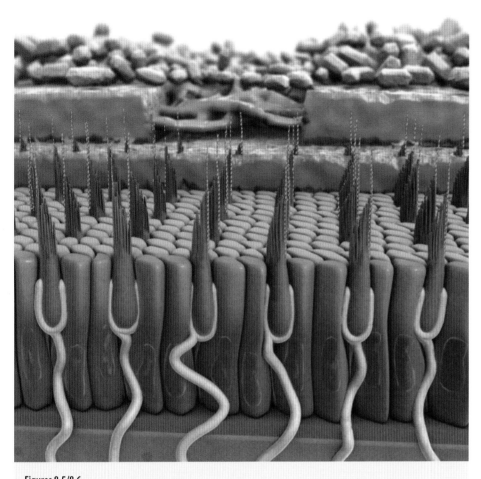

Figures 8.5/8.6

Specialized mechanoreceptors within the inner ear's passageways. The ampullary cupulae (center of Figure 8.5, facing page) sense the movement of fluid caused by rotational movement, while two types of sensitive hair cells (Figure 8.6, brown and green) sense the inertia of the stone-like otoliths (top of Figure 8.6 above, grey) in linear movements.

Be sure you are very comfortable in your own body as well. Your ability to stay relaxed and extremely stable will be key to the effectiveness of the technique, as you will be holding your client's head up for several minutes. If your client is much larger than you, or has a particularly heavy head, this means you will need to experiment with hand and body positions to find variations that work for you. Although I typically use the hand position pictured in Figure 8.7 (seated with one hand under the head, forearm on the table, and my elbows close in to my sides), some practitioners find it easier to stand, cross their arms behind the client's head palm-down, with the right palm on the client's left shoulder and the left palm on the client's right shoulder, and lift using their legs and body, rather than with just the arms.

Whatever position you choose, make sure your supporting point of contact is physically beneath (posterior to) your client's head. The supporting sensation of touch on the back of the head feels safe and reassuring, and helps encourage further release and relaxation.

Once both you and your client are comfortable in this lifted-head position, begin to gradually lower the head, ever so slowly, bit by infinitesimal bit. At this point, we come to the most important part of the technique: as you lower the head in super-slow motion, feel for your client's ability to let the head go, every millimeter of the way. If you are sensitive and slow enough, you will feel small variations in the perceived weight of your client's head. If your client's head seems to get lighter, you are lowering faster than his or her ability to release. If this is the case, stop, back up a millimeter, and wait for your client to surrender the head again.

Avoid casual chatter that might distract your client; however, verbal cues that help your client focus can be invaluable. If you wait for a while with no release, try a gentle verbal prompt such

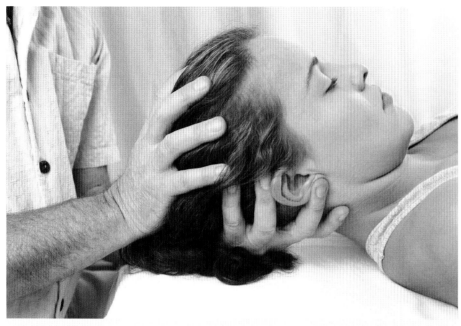

Figure 8.7

In the Vestibular Orienting Technique, the head is lowered extremely slowly, while the practitioner feels for the slightest hint of the client holding or bracing the head. When these responses are encountered, the lowering is stopped or slightly reversed, while the client is instructed to breathe, relax, and allow an even heavier head. If vertigo is encountered, keeping the eyes open can help prevent or alleviate dizziness.

as: "Just allow your head to be heavy," or "On your next exhale, let your head release a little more." Some clients will actively push their heads downwards towards the table in response to these prompts. Patiently cue these clients towards release and relaxation, rather than pushing or exerting effort. Asking for small, slow, active eye movements, or conscious exhaling can also help when release is difficult.

Though it requires patience and sensitivity, this technique is procedurally very simple. So, how does it affect the vestibular system? The head and neck's orienting reflexes are initiated by vestibular signaling. The small fluctuations in your client's ability to let the head go are signs that his or her vestibular system and brain are renegotiating the habitual muscle tension related to orienting and righting the head. Your super-slow head lowering provides just enough rotational stimuli to evoke a vestibular response. The places where you might feel your client subtly stiffen may correspond to angles and positions where the inner ears' semicircular canals are hypersensitive, or where they might be habitually accustomed to raising the "bracing needed!" alarm.

Waiting, or subtly backing up in the places where you feel this slight stiffening allows a client's nervous system to accommodate a new threshold of activation. By waiting and relaxing into each place where the slight stiffening starts, your client's nervous system increases its adaptive range; this resets the stimulus thresholds that previously resulted in bracing. Your client's nervous system is also being reminded that everything is actually okay; that nothing bad happens in this position—the head does not fall over, get whipped around, or experience pain. These are examples of some of the subconscious catastrophic expectations that may be coupled with relaxing into particular head and neck positions. Of course, not everyone's neck bracing is related to body memories of physical trauma; sometimes, it is simply hard to let the head go. Tension, stress, eye or jaw strain, postural habit, illness or, as described earlier, support or stability deficits elsewhere in the body, can all contribute to vestibular reactivity and bracing patterns.

As mentioned, this technique can often help clients who have pre-existing dizziness or vertigo, as long as special care is taken to keep the eyes open (since vertigo, like motion sickness, is often activated by contradictory information from the inner ears and the eyes). It is also important not to lift the head so far or fast that the dizziness is worsened. Once activated, vertigo may need some time to subside before attempting the technique again. A small minority of clients with vertigo will not be able to tolerate any head lifting or holding. This technique would be contraindicated for these clients, as it would be for clients with a very recent or serious neck injury.

Lowering the head in the sagittal plane, as described here, stimulates two of the inner ears' three canals related to rotational motion (the anterior and posterior semicircular canals).

The third horizontal semicircular canal can be engaged with slow side-to-side rolling of the head, again feeling for your client's ability to release the head at each step of the way.

Another variation is to carefully work with the client's head off the edge of the table, or to use a drop-table to continue lowering the head posteriorly past its anatomical position. This allows you to work with a larger range in the sagittal plane. However, keep in mind that having your client's head off the end of a table violates our earlier perceived-safety principle of making sure there is something underneath the head to support it. In addition, neck hyperextension itself can aggravate some neck conditions, so keep the neck long, use this variation with care, and use it only with relatively healthy clients.

Whichever variation you choose, once you have lowered the head to the table, you have finished this technique and are ready to move on in your session. Patience is key. You can easily perform this technique too quickly, but I do not think that it can be completed too slowly. Taking a full five or even 10 minutes to lower the head once will be time quite well spent.

See video of the Vestibular Orienting Technique at www.a-t.tv/na02

Key points: Vestibular Orienting Technique

Indications include:

- Vertigo.
- Mild to moderate hot whiplash, as long as technique is calming and comfortable (contraindicated if supine position or head lifting increase discomfort).
- Sympathetic autonomic nervous system activation.
- Anxiety, tension, disquiet.

Purpose

- Calm sympathetic nervous system activation, especially when related to balance difficulties or instability.
- Increase the nervous system's adaptive range (raising the thresholds at which bracing postural reflexes are triggered).

Instructions

1. Lift your supine client's head into comfortable neck flexion, being sure to provide ample support to the back of the head.
2. Make sure you're comfortable, stable, and relaxed.
3. Very slowly, lower the head back towards the table.
4. Pause whenever you feel tension or bracing; wait for your client to once again surrender the head's weight.
5. Cue client to relax, breathe, release the weight of the head.
6. If vertigo or nausea increase, return to last position of comfort. Have client keep eyes open. Wait for symptoms to subside before continuing.
7. Take your time. This technique should take at least several minutes to complete.

Variations

- Explore cervical rotation (head on the table) in the same way.
- On clients who are able to (those without acute injuries, instability, or strong vertigo), allow the head and neck to drop below the level of the table, into slight cervical extension. Keep neck long.

References

[1] Sadler, T.W. (2012) *Langman's medical embryology.* 12th ed. Philadelphia: Wolters Kluwer Health/Lippincott Williams & Wilkins. p. 321–327.

[2] Richard, W. et al. (2005) Efficacy of the Epley maneuver for posterior canal BPPV: A long-term, controlled study of 81 patients. *Ear, Nose, & Throat Journal.* 84(1). p. 22–25.

[3] Yates, B.J. et al. (2005) The effects of vestibular system lesions on autonomic regulation: Observations, mechanisms, and clinical implications. *Journal of Vestibular Research.* 15. p. 119–129.

[4] Feldenkrais, M. (1979) *Explorers of Humankind.* San Francisco: Harper and Row.

Picture credits

Figures 8.1, 8.2, 8.3, 8.4, 8.5, and 8.6 Primal Pictures, used by permission. Figure 8.7 Advanced-Trainings.com.

Study Guide

The Vestibular System

1 **What is one of the effects of vestibular system stimulation mentioned in the text?**

a parasympathetic (rest and repair) ANS activation
b sympathetic (fight or flight) ANS activation
c decreased muscular tension throughout the body
d lower blood pressure

2 **What is one thing the text suggest the client can do to reduce any dizziness during the Vestibular Orienting Technique?**

a keep the eyes open
b close the eyes
c hold a deep breath
d think about something pleasant

3 **According to the chapter, what does the vestibular system sense?**

a head movement
b position of the head in space
c joint position
d gravity

4 **What is the suggested speed used for lowering the head in the Vestibular Orienting Technique?**

a slow
b super slow
c moderate
d no speed was suggested

5 **What is the practitioner feeling for in the Vestibular Orienting Technique?**

a the client's ability to let the pelvis be heavy
b the range of cervical flexion
c the client's ability to let the head be heavy
d the range of cervical extension

For Answer Keys, visit www.Advanced-Trainings.com/v2key/

Hot Whiplash

For hands-on practitioners, there is good and bad news about whiplash. The bad news first: whiplash injuries puzzle and befuddle manual therapists. How do we know this? Not only do we hear this regularly from practitioners in our Advanced Myofascial Techniques courses, but when we surveyed 100 experienced practitioners on the conditions they would most like to learn more about, whiplash was the most frequently mentioned issue.

More bad news: Whiplash is common. Although estimates vary, several sources cite about 1.8 million new cases of whiplash per year in the US alone (1).

Whiplash is also complicated—sufferers experience a wide array of physical, neurological, and psychobiological symptoms, which may not appear until weeks or months after the original injury. Symptoms can persist for months or years and, for a significant number of sufferers, get worse over time. One study published in the European Spine Journal found that during the first and second years following a motor vehicle accident, the symptoms of over 20 percent of whiplash sufferers worsened (2). Although there have been hundreds of studies on whiplash, and more are conducted each year, there is widespread disagreement on diagnosis, treatment, and even terminology;[1] most interventions for whiplash injury are considered "medically unproven" (3) and the reasons for whiplash's intractability are only beginning to be understood. The psychobiological impact of whiplash has long been recognized, and significant numbers of whiplash sufferers experience anxiety, depression, or symptoms similar to post-traumatic stress (4). What is more, whiplash patients can be involved in legal or insurance difficulties, which may complicate and even hinder recovery (5).

If this wasn't enough bad news, manual practitioners observe that whiplash symptoms can worsen after bodywork—almost as if their hands-on work had opened a Pandora's Box of pain, soreness, and spasm. The aim of this chapter is to help you prevent this.

Despite all of the above, there is good news about whiplash. In spite of its complexity, hands-on body therapy can help. Skilled practitioners are getting very good results by using soft tissue release together with neurologically based approaches. Gentle encouragement of motility, such as that provided by sensitive and competent manual therapy, in combination with moderate activity, is one of the most widely agreed-upon conventional treatments for whiplash. (Immobilization and cervical collars, once the most common treatment, are now rarely used, as they have been observed to produce more problems than they resolve (6).) An increasing understanding of the effects of trauma on the nervous system is expanding manual therapists' ability to help clients whose symptoms were previously only aggravated by hands-on work.

The effects of whiplash

The effects of whiplash range from mild to severe, can change over time, and may include any or all of the following:

- Tissue damage at the sites of injury, from local overstretching or micro-tearing of fascia, muscle, or nerve tissues, typically in the neck, shoulders, and back.
- Harmonic forces in the body, bracing reactions, and fascial connections can cause tissue injury and inflammation in unexpected, non-local areas anywhere in the body, such as the ribcage, limbs, or pelvis.

---

1 The term "whiplash" was first used to describe cervical injuries in 1928 by orthopedic surgeon Harold Crowe, and is subject to some controversy. Physical medicine texts variously prefer the terms "acceleration-deceleration injury," "hyperflexion-hyperextension injury," or "cervical strain-sprain injury."

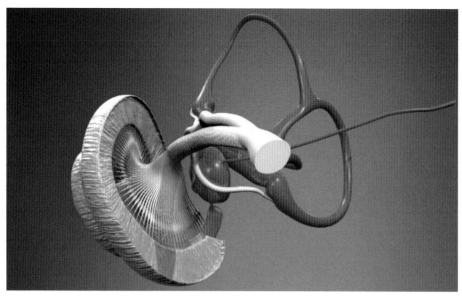

Figure 9.1

The structures of the inner ear. Dizziness and vertigo after whiplash can be exacerbated by loss of adaptability in the neck. This can limit the body's ability to position the head and adapt to stimulus from the balance mechanisms of the inner ear's semicircular canals (blue, right).

- Instability or weakness from tissue damage, and from dissociation of the muscle spindle/Golgi postural reflex relationships in the injured muscles, resulting from overstretch (7).
- Restricted motion as a result of either acute muscle spasticity/splinting reflexes, or from chronically adhered and shortened connective tissues, including the tissues around articulations.
- Pain, anywhere in the body. Causes may include direct tissue injury, neurologically referred pain, peripheral or central sensitization, or autonomically associated pain, e.g. post-traumatic headaches.
- Vertigo (dizziness) and balance impairment: cervical instability can result in splinting and fixing of the neck and head (especially by the suboccipital muscles), which reduces the adaptive capacity of the vestibular system (Figure 9.1). (See Chapter 8, *The Vestibular System*.) Post-traumatic vertigo is also postulated to be related to sympathetic nervous system imbalance (8).
- Sympathetic (fight or flight) activation of the autonomic nervous system (ANS) from the trauma of the incident itself; from direct injury to sympathetic nerve fibers in the neck (Figure 9.2) (9) or from ongoing sympathetic stimulation from vestibular and balance impairment. Symptoms can include sleeplessness, headaches, anxiety, or depression.

Some of the more severe effects of whiplash, such as prolonged anxiety or depression, obviously necessitate referral to a qualified specialist. In particular, clients with vertigo, nausea, or ocular discomfort that worsen with head movement should be referred to a physician for evaluation before any manipulation is performed, as this can indicate vascular, ligament, or spinal cord issues. These examples aside, many of the effects of whiplash are well within our power to ameliorate.

	Hot	Cold
Time Since Injury	Usually recent.	At least 3–6 weeks since injury.
Symptoms	Pain, instability, spasm; guarded or careful movement.	Pain, immobility, inflexibility; restricted or stiff movement.
Mobility Restriction	Muscular hyper-tonus (spasm).	Fascial hardening; ligamentous and articular restrictions.
Tissue Quality	Inflamed, puffy, slippery; sometimes soft, sometimes hyper-toned; touch is often painful.	Hard, dense, rigid, especially at deep levels. Can be insensitive to light touch.
Goals	Calm unresolved fight or flight activation; encourage subtle motility; broaden client's focus beyond injury.	Release tissue restrictions; restore lost gross mobility.
Strategy	Work primarily with nervous system; work within client's range of active motility; address myofascial restrictions only away from injured areas.	Work with myofascial restrictions and movement barriers to restore mobility, both locally and globally.
Metaphor	Imagine working on a bare nervous system: use delicate, slow, gentle touch.	Imagine melting frozen tissue with the warmth, pressure, and patience of your touch.

Table 9.1 Hot and cold whiplash compared.

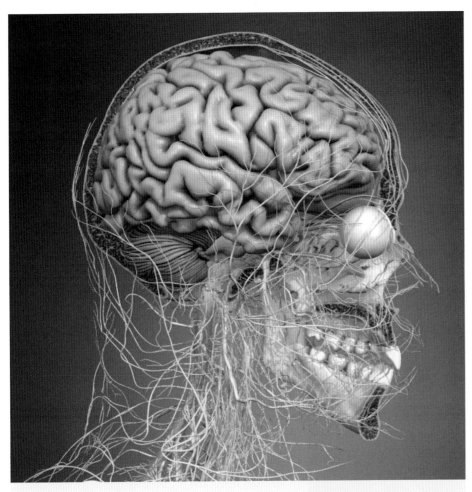

Figure 9.2

It can be helpful when working with hot whiplash to imagine working on a bare nervous system. Hyperextension injury to the cervical portion of the sympathetic trunks of prevertebral ganglia (green, anterior neck) is thought to contribute to vertigo and other autonomic symptoms associated with whiplash.

Hot and cold whiplash

Metaphorically, it can be helpful to think of whiplash as having either "hot" or "cold" qualities. A recent whiplash (less than 3–6 weeks) will tend to show more hot qualities, while cold whiplash is typically older (although older whiplash can also be hot, or can turn hot if reinjured or worked insensitively). Table 9.1 summarizes differences between these two phases of the body's response. Although you can see elements of both hot and cold whiplash in the same client, it is important to differentiate the way you work with each type of symptom, as hot and cold whiplash can respond very differently to the same interventions.

Hot whiplash is distinguished by being sensitive, fragile, and reactive, as the fight or flight responses of the autonomic nervous system are still aroused. The head and neck are typically immobilized by muscular spasm or hypertonus since the postural reflexes recruit muscular tension to provide the inherent structural stability that has been compromised by the injury. Because of tissue damage, inflammation will be a factor in a recent or unresolved whiplash. The tissue in injured areas will feel softer or puffy to your gentle palpation (though not always literally hot). Your client may respond to direct touch with guarding, uneasiness, or pain, which further increases sympathetic activation.

In contrast, cold whiplash is typically older, less autonomically reactive, and restricted at the ligamentous or joint level (as opposed to being primarily immobilized by muscular spasm). Cold whiplash is characterized by stubborn, dense, hardened tissue deep around the joints. Hot whiplash often becomes cold (restricted) once initial tissue damage has begun to heal; cold whiplash can become hot (re-activated) if worked too quickly or aggressively. We'll focus on hot whiplash in this chapter, and cold whiplash in the next.

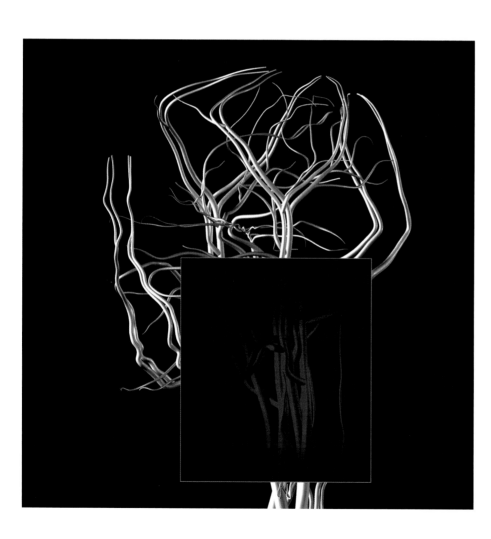

Working with hot whiplash

When working with hot whiplash, our primary goal is to calm our client's autonomic activation, before trying to work with any tissue restrictions. To get a sense of this, imagine that you're working on an exposed, unprotected central nervous system. In a way, you are—after a traumatic event, our ability to filter out or tolerate intense experience decreases, leaving us feeling vulnerable and unshielded. How would you touch a client who was nothing but a bare brain and spinal cord? Hopefully, very delicately and carefully—this is the ideal way to approach a recent or hot whiplash.

As sympathetic re-activation can happen by working either too long, too fast, or too deeply, it is important to pace your work. Try to do shorter sessions with small, supportive, calming interventions. Watch to see how your client responds to your work, both within and between sessions. Gradually increase duration, scope, or depth as your client is ready—you can always work a little more next time, but it is hard to take back your work, if you've done too much.

Work elsewhere in the body, before and after approaching any injured or painful areas. This broadens your client's awareness beyond their places of injury and pain. Use the metaphor of a tangle of yarn or string: you wouldn't go right the tightest part of a tangle and start pulling (Figure 9.5). Instead, work at the periphery, gently and patiently loosening the overall pattern.

Encourage motility, instead of trying to mobilize. Use your client's gentle active motion (i.e. motility) to restore subtle movement to spastic areas, instead of applying passive manipulation, stretching, or direct release techniques (which can mobilize, but could re-aggravate). Breath, active exploration of range of motion, and even micromovements will help restore disrupted reflexes and prevent tissue adhesion. Direct work

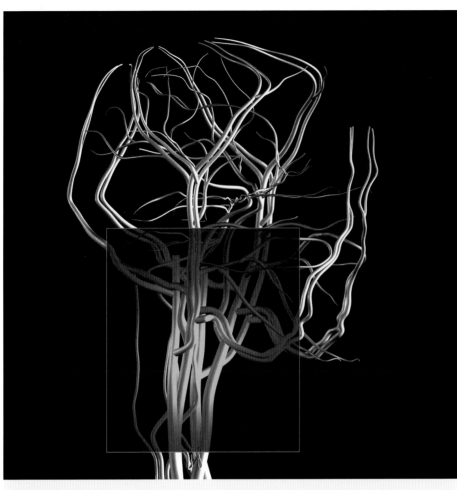

Figures 9.3/9.4

Metaphorically, whiplash can be thought of as having hot and cold qualities. Though a whiplash injury typically progresses from hot to cold over time, even an older whiplash can exhibit hot qualities, particularly if reinjured or worked too aggressively.

with gross movement barriers or tissue restrictions come later, once muscular splinting has subsided and injured tissues are less inflamed.

There are many ways to work that accomplish these goals; much of what you probably already know about relaxing and calming can be extremely effective when applied with the above considerations in mind. A specific technique that incorporates these principles is the Breath Motility Technique.

Breath Motility Technique

Breath has the power to calm the nervous system, to catalyze lost motility, and to bring proprioceptive awareness to the otherwise healthy regions that have been eclipsed by the painful areas.

Begin by asking your client to take a normal breath, and look to see where the thorax moves the most with inhalation. Using a soft, receptive touch, sandwich that place, front and back, between your hands, as in Figures 9.6 and 9.7. Whether the breath starts in the belly, diaphragm, or chest, ask your client to allow the space between your hands to fill gently with a normal breath. Note: We don't say, "push the breath between my hands," or even "breathe here." Those imperatives will evoke a more efforted response than the invitation to simply "allow" the breath to fill between your hands. Our aims are: calm the autonomic responses; induce gentle active movement in places that have lost it; and increase proprioception. Try it in your own body—a forcibly inhaled breath doesn't accomplish those aims as well as a breath that you simply allow to come in on its own. You'll be able to palpate the difference in your client's breath too. Continue to coach and encourage your client until the breath is effortless, and it is tangibly clear to each of you that the breath is moving in between your hands, both front and back.

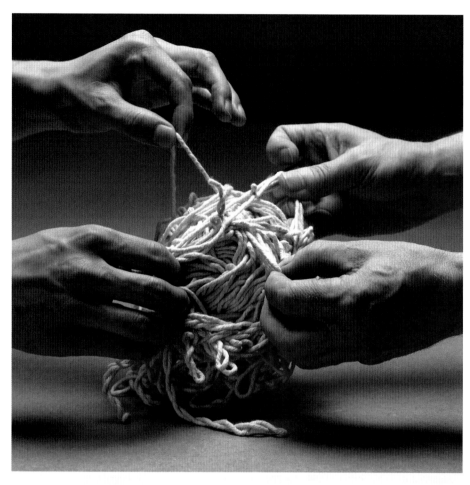

Figure 9.5

Whether hot or cold, approach whiplash in the same way you might gradually untangle a stubborn knot in a rope or cord: avoid pulling at the tightest places; instead, tease the tangle apart by loosening the periphery, and gradually work your way in.

See video of the Breath Motility Technique at www.a-t.tv/ad05

When both you and your client feel the breath moving in an area, move to a new place nearby, and repeat. Keep the pacing even, and the breath normal. Deep or fast breathing, especially high in the chest, will increase sympathetic activity, rather than calm it. Continue to get agreement from your client about his or her ability to sense the breath in each new area. Stay encouraging, interested, and focused. If it is difficult for your client to feel the breath in a new place, or if you don't feel it with your hands, return to the last spot where it was clear, and move out gradually from there. Repeat this pattern with the entire thorax and abdomen, on both left and right sides. Take at least 10 minutes for this technique, although allowing longer for it would be time well spent. This simple technique could be the bulk of an entire session, which would leave your client feeling more settled and relaxed.

Incidentally, if you notice that your client's movement is guarded or painful, you may want to perform this technique with your client seated, rather than supine. Seated work in general can be very helpful, if the act of lying down is painful or difficult.

These ideas should help you avoid the "Pandora's Box" effect of making whiplash pain worse with inappropriately deep or direct work. In the next chapter, we'll share tips for recognizing and working with the chronic, stubborn patterns typical of cold whiplash, where deep and direct work can be just what is needed.

Key points: Breath Motility Technique

Indications include:

- Signs of sympathetic (fight or flight) autonomic activation.
- Recent (less than 3–6 weeks) or "hot" whiplash.
- Immobility due to muscle spasm or splinting.
- Also useful whenever increased proprioception of breath is indicated.

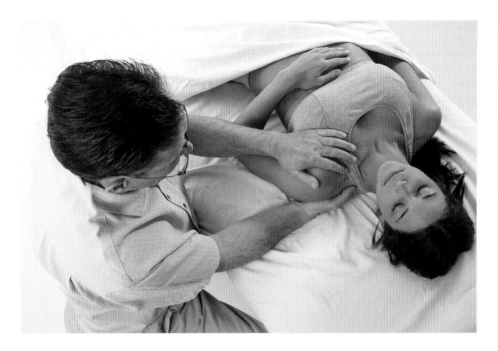

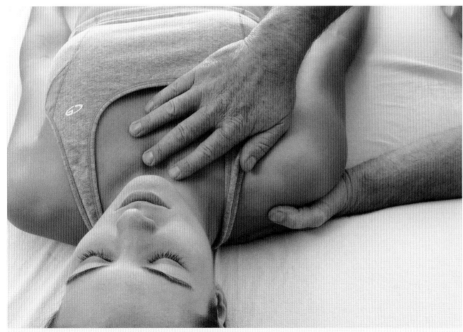

Figures 9.6/9.7

The Breath Motility Technique is used when initiating work with hot whiplash, in order to soothe the nervous system, increase motility, and broaden the client's proprioceptive awareness beyond painful areas.

Purpose

- Increase proprioception of breath.
- Calm autonomic nervous system.
- Encourage breath motility in all directions.
- (In pain or acute injury,) increase awareness of non-painful areas of the body.

Instructions

1. Observe client's breath, noting areas of diminished movement.
2. Gently "sandwich" this area between your hands.
3. Invite the client to allow breath into this area, using normal, un-efforted breathing.
4. Give verbal feedback and encouragement. Make sure both you and your client feel breath movement.
5. If difficult, begin in another area where breath motility is obvious to the client, then move into areas of less movement.
6. Take your time, working any areas of diminished motility in the thorax and abdomen (or elsewhere in the body).

References

[1] Estimates of whiplash prevalence ranges from a low of 120,000 new cases annually (quoted in "Prevalence and Incidence Statistics for Whiplash," www.rightdiagnosis.com/w/whiplash/prevalence.htm. [Accessed December 2015]), to a high estimate of 1,800,000 new annual cases (as cited in several chiropractic sources, including Croft, Arthur C. (2009) *Facts Concerning Whiplash Injuries*, Spine Research Institute of San Diego http://www.docstoc.com/docs/3822558/Facts-Concerning-Whiplash-Injuries-by-Arthur-C-Croft-DC-MS#. [Accessed December 2015]

[2] A study published in the European Spine Journal found that during the period of time between the first and second years following a motor vehicle accident, over 20 percent had symptoms worsen: Olivegren, H., Jerkvall, N., Hagstrom, Y., and Carlsson, J. (1999) The long-term prognosis of whiplash-associated disorders (WAD). *European Spine Journal*. 8(5). p. 366–370.

[3] Spitzer, W.O., Skovron, M.L., Salmi, L.R., Cassidy, J.D., Duranceau, J., Suissa, S., and Zeiss, E. (1995) Scientific monograph of the Quebec Task Force on Whiplash-Associated Disorders: Redefining "whiplash" and its management. *Spine* (Phila Pa 1976). 1995 Apr 15; 20(8 Suppl):1S–73S.

[4] In 1961, physician Robert Munro wrote: "In its pure form and when rightly diagnosed, the symptoms of 'whiplash' injury are those of cervical muscular spasm often complicated by neurosis." From: Munro, R. (1961) Treatment of fractures and dislocations of the cervical spine. *New England Journal of Medicine*. 264. p. 573–582.

[5] Statistically, whiplash sufferers with workers' compensation claims or lawsuits have significantly worse outcomes than those who do not. In fact, in studies designed to judge the efficacy of interventions, investigators often exclude such patients or report their results separately. From: Brian Grottkau, M.D., writing in the *New England Journal of Medicine* (348, no. 14 (April 3, 2003): 1413–1414) about Andrew Malleson's book *Whiplash and Other Useful Illnesses.*

[6] Use of immobilization and cervical collars after whiplash injury have been observed to produce temporomandibular dysfunction, joint adhesions, muscle atrophy, and myofascial trigger points. Lowe, W. (2003) Assess & address: Whiplash. *Massage Magazine,* 104 (July/August).

[7] Cailliet, R. (1991) *Neck and Arm Pain.* Philadelphia, PA: F.A. Davis Company. p. 88.

[8] Cailliet, R. (1991) ibid., p. 112.

[9] Cailliet, R. (1991) ibid., p. 112.

Picture credits

Figures 9.1 and 9.2 Primal Pictures, used by permission.

Figures 9.3, 9.4, and 9.5 Thinkstock.

Figures 9.6 and 9.7 Advanced-Trainings.com.

Study Guide

Hot Whiplash

1 **What is listed as our primary goal in working with hot whiplash?**

a reducing pain
b reducing inflammation
c reducing tissue restrictions
d reducing autonomic activation

2 **Which of the following does the text associate with cold whiplash (more than with hot whiplash)?**

a muscle spasm
b tissue inflammation
c restricted articular movement
d sympathetic ANS activation

3 **Which of the following does the text associate with hot whiplash (more than with cold whiplash)?**

a muscle spasm
b articular restrictions
c tissue inflexibility
d restricted movement

4 **According to the text, which of the whiplash symptoms listed below would be a cause for physician referral?**

a restricted neck/head motion
b increased nausea with head movement
c micro-tearing of tissues
d tissue instability or weakness

5 **According to the text, how should myofascial restrictions be address in a hot whiplash?**

a with direct techniques
b gently at the injury site
c away from the injury site
d not until 3–6 weeks

For Answer Keys, visit www.Advanced-Trainings.com/v2key/

Cold Whiplash

In the previous chapter, we discussed how whiplash can have metaphorically "hot" and "cold" phases, and some approaches for working with hot patterns. In this chapter, I will describe two techniques from Advanced-Trainings.com's Advanced Myofascial Techniques repertory that are particularly effective for working with cold whiplash. I will also share some of our instructors' advice and best practices for strategizing whiplash sessions.

Here is a brief review of our hot/cold distinction: hot whiplash is usually (but not always) more recent, generally within six weeks of the injury. Hot whiplash is characterized by sympathetic nervous system ("fight or flight") arousal, inflamed and hypersensitive tissues (anywhere in the body), and immobilization and guarding via muscular contraction and spasm. Once some time has passed, an older but still unresolved whiplash can show the "cold" pattern of hard, dense connective tissue restrictions (vs. muscular spasm), especially deep around the joints, which also limits mobility.

Hot whiplash needs to be worked very carefully to avoid increasing the tissue inflammation and further aggravating the client's autonomic arousal. Cold whiplash can usually be approached more directly, however we're not out of the woods yet as cold whiplash can easily be re-activated into a hot pattern if worked too much, too deeply, or too fast. Go slowly until you can assess how your client is responding.

The primary goals in working with hot whiplash are to calm the aggravated nervous system responses and to encourage whole-body *motility* (self-generated movement), which helps minimize connective tissue scarring and layer adhesion (1). Only when a whiplash has progressed to the cold stage do we add the additional primary goal of restoring local *mobility* (the ability to move or be moved) by directly addressing movement and tissue restrictions.[1]

Cervical Core/Sleeve Technique

As shown in Figure 10.1, a sudden backward acceleration of the head, such as that caused by a rear-end impact or a fall, can violently overextend and injure the soft tissues of the anterior neck (amongst other structures). Once the inflammation and guarding of the hot stage has diminished, and the rest of the body has been prepared (see the Whiplash Tips, p104), you can begin addressing the tissues of the anterior neck by working the neck's outer "sleeve" — the superficial layers of cervical fascia and the underlying sternocleidomastoids (SCM).

Since we're beginning with superficial layers, the tool we'll use is the soft fist, as the drier texture of the skin on the dorsum of the hand is better suited for superficial work than the palm. Rather than a hard, closed fist, a soft fist is open, easy, and relaxed, and both the fingers and thumb are out and comfortable (Figures 10.2 and 10.3). It is important to keep the wrist and metacarpals aligned with the forearm—this protects your wrist from strain and compression, and allows you to work with less effort, making your touch more sensitive.

Using the proximal knuckles of your soft fist, gently catch the outer layers of the neck, just anterior and superficial to the SCM belly. We don't use oil or lotion at this stage, as we'll need to use the gentle friction of the soft fist to differentiate and free up the tissue layers we're working.

Take up any slack in the outer wrappings of the neck by moving the outer layers posteriorly. There are delicate structures in the neck, so be sure you're

---

1 In both hot and cold whiplash there are often additional secondary symptom-specific goals, such as headache relief in the case of hot whiplash (Chapter 9), or easing the jaw tension and pain that can accompany either hot or cold whiplash (Chapter 16).

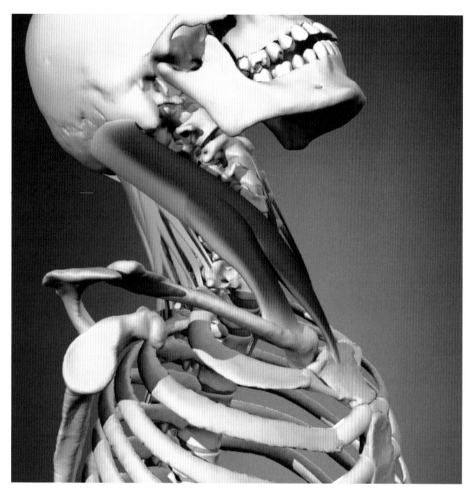

Figure 10.1

In a rear-end impact or a backwards fall, the head and neck can be thrown backwards into hyperextension, overstretching and injuring soft tissues of the shoulders, chest, spine, and anterior neck, such as the sternocleidomastoid (red).

staying on superficial tissues only. Think about just catching the outer collar of a turtleneck sweater, without putting any pressure on the deeper structures, or without pulling the "collar" too tightly across the front of the throat. Your client should be comfortable—if he or she feels that you're pressing too deeply, or pulling too much on the front of the throat, readjust your pressure, layer, and/or direction until there is no discomfort.

After carefully taking up the slack of the outer layers, ask your client to slowly turn his or her head away from the side you're working. Your working hand is static, so any sliding on the skin's surface is initiated by the client's movement and tissue release. Make sure your client's movement is slow and focused—"muscling through" the movement won't help your client learn an easier way of moving, and might even cause you both to miss the cues that keep your pressure safe. Optimally, your client's head and neck should stay aligned, moving around the longitudinal axis of the spine, rather than rolling off to the side. In Figure 10.2, my right hand is gently guiding my client's head with this alignment in mind. You can repeat this anchoring and turning in two or three places between the base of the neck and the base of the skull, and at the slightly deeper layer of the SCM; then repeat on the opposite side.

This technique can also serve as a great finishing move: Ida Rolf PhD (the originator or Rolfing® structural integration) often used a similar technique to make sure her client's neck was adaptable, long, and free at the end of her sessions.

Key points: Cervical Core/Sleeve Technique

Indications include:
- Cold whiplash.
- Neck mobility issues, tension, or pain.
- TMJ or jaw issues.

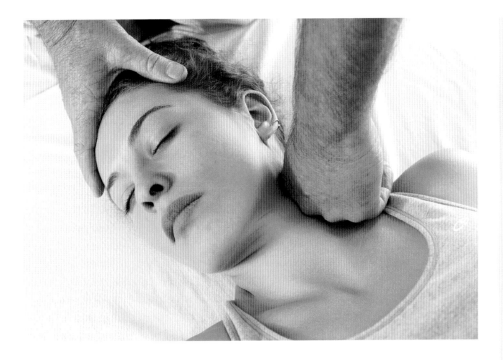

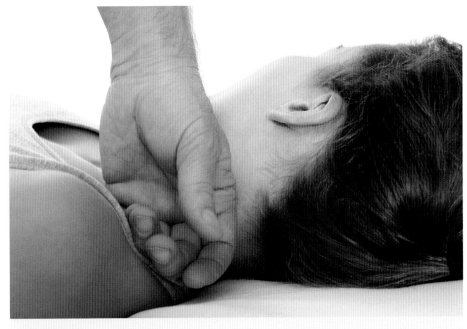

Figures 10.2/10.3

Cervical Core/Sleeve Technique: Gently use the backside of a soft, open hand to ease the outer layers of the neck posteriorly. Do not put any pressure on the underlying structures of the throat and neck—the styloid process, lymph nodes, carotid artery, and vagus nerve, amongst other sensitive structures, are all in this region and merit special care.

Purpose
- Differentiate superficial and deep fascial layers (sleeve/core).
- Restore any diminished cervical mobility.
- Preparation for deeper neck work.
- Ensuring neck adaptability when finishing a session.

Instructions
Standing at the head or side of your supine client,
1. Use a soft fist just anterior and superficial to the SCM to take up any slack in the outer fascial layers of the neck;
2. Use client's slow and deliberate active rotation to slide cervical fascial layers under your static touch; feel for layer-to-layer differentiation.

Be sure to stay on superficial layers to avoid discomfort or injury to deeper neck structures.

Movements
- Slow neck rotation, away from the side being worked.
- Maintain longitudinal alignment through the neck (instead of rolling or sidebending).

Lateral Cervical Translation Technique

The deepest soft-tissue structures of the neck, such as the zygapophyseal (or facet) joint capsules and ligaments, can be primary sources of pain and movement restriction long after a whiplash injury has occurred (2). Once the inflammation of the original injury has settled, restoring mobility to these deep structures can provide significant relief.

Lateral translation refers to side-to-side movement of one vertebra in relation to another. In order to check for movement restrictions at the facet joints, we'll feel for the freedom of this movement at each vertebra, since the other movements of the neck—flexion/extension, rotation, and lateral bending—will be affected by the same connective tissues that restrict translation.

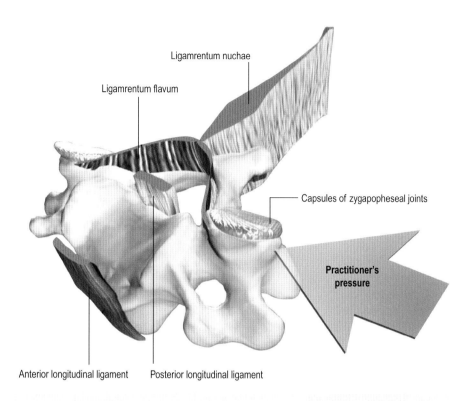

Ligamrentum nuchae

Ligamrentum flavum

Capsules of zygapopheseal joints

Practitioner's pressure

Anterior longitudinal ligament

Posterior longitudinal ligament

Figure 10.4

The ligamentous structures surrounding a cervical vertebra. The purple arrow indicates placement and direction of gentle pressure in the Translation Technique.

Any of several deep structures can be involved: the facet joint capsules, the ligamentum flavum, as well as the small intertransverse ligaments and muscles (Figures 10.4 and 10.9). These very deep structures are either difficult or impossible to palpate directly, but assessing cervical translation allows us to effectively locate and release any of the structures that are restricting free motion.

To perform the technique, begin by gently feeling for the boniest lateral projections of the cervical vertebrae, at and just posterior to the lateral midline of the cervical spine. These projections are the small transverse processes, and the articular processes just behind them. Together, these lateral protrusions form a relatively wide platform for your touch (Figure 10.4, and 10.9, arrow). Don't worry about being too exact—simply feel for the most prominent, non-painful bony lateral projection.

Next, using the broad, soft pads of several fingers on these projections, feel for straight side-to-side movement of each cervical vertebra. Your touch should stay broad and soft; avoid poking. Although you'll want to feel for isolated movement at each individual vertebra, do this by leaving the head on the table (neck neither flexed nor extended), and moving the head laterally together with the entire cervical spine above (cephalad to) the vertebra you're assessing (Figure 10.5), as if moving a stack of coins or poker chips (Figure 10.6): move the single coin (vertebra) together with the entire stack of coins above that point.

Assess the entire length of the neck before trying to release individual restrictions; assess each vertebra in turn, for both left and right translation. Be thorough by starting at the base of the neck, and working upwards. Typically, you'll find that some vertebrae translate easier to one side than the other. If there's been a whiplash injury, these left-right differences are often quite pronounced.

Beginning with one of the most restricted vertebrae, encourage easier translation in the restricted direction by gently but firmly pressing that vertebra in the more difficult direction. Using this vertebra as a fulcrum, simultaneously side-bend the neck the opposite direction. For example, if a vertebra is difficult to translate left, press that vertebra left (Figures 10.7 and 10.9, arrows), and sidebend the neck right at the fulcrum point (Figure 10.8). Why sidebend, if we're checking translation? Sidebending asks for the facets to either open or close (depending on whether they are on the concave or convex side of the sidebend), and the facets are the same structures that are likely limiting any restricted translation. This sidebending/fulcrum approach is an effective way to focus the pressure right at the joints that are most likely restricting the translated motion.

The example above describes a direct approach—in other words, you'll encourage the restricted vertebra to translate more in the direction it doesn't easily go, by sidebending the neck around your firm-yet-sensitive, broad-yet-specific touch. Since we're asking for deep, ligamentous change, you'll need to be patient and wait for the body to respond—for four to six breaths, at least—until you feel a gradual softening or easing of the hard restriction. Then, recheck. If you've been specific enough, gentle enough, and patient enough, you'll feel more movement in the previously restricted direction. Repeat this procedure for each translation restriction you found.

Some Variations of the Lateral Cervical Translation Technique

1. The above procedure is described with the neck in a neutral position, that is, neither flexed nor extended. By passively flexing or extending the neck slightly during assessment and release, you'll sometimes find even more restrictions, or get results unavailable in the neutral neck position.

2. Occasionally, an indirect release is helpful with a particularly stubborn area. This involves

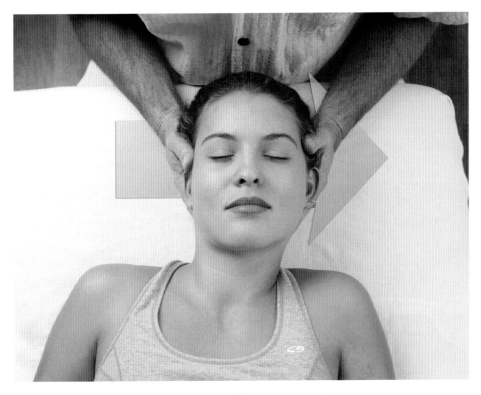

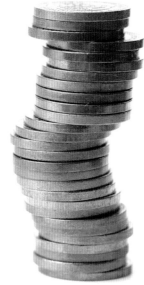

Figures 10.5/10.6

To assess cervical translation, cradle and move the head together with the vertebrae above the individual vertebra being assessed. In this case, left translation of C4 is being assessed. Not visible from this angle are the finger pads isolating the translation movement at a single cervical vertebra (as in Figure 10.7). It can help to imagine the vertebrae like a stack of coins; hold and move the whole stack above the individual "coin" that you want to assess.

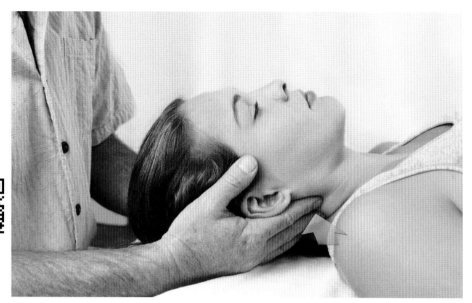

See video of the Lateral Cervical Translation at www.a-t.tv/nb05

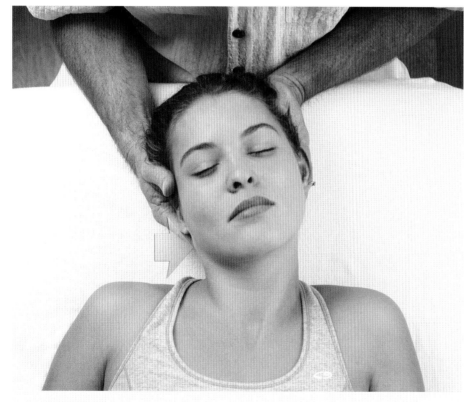

Figures 10.7/10.8

To release translation restrictions, gently sidebend the neck around the fulcrum of your finger pressure (arrow) and wait for the subtle softening of a ligamentous response. Pictured here is a direct release for a vertebra that resists left translation.

gently sidebending the neck in the opposite direction to that described above—in other words, taking the restricted vertebra further into its easier direction, instead of into the barrier. This can help ease into the restriction, and is particularly useful if there is still guarding or sensitivity. However, we've found that direct work, as long as you are patient and sensitive, is effective for the majority of cases.

Key points: Lateral Cervical Translation Technique

Indications include:

- Cold whiplash.
- Neck mobility issues, tension, or pain.
- Tension headaches.
- Torticollis.

Purpose

- Assess and restore any lost cervical facet joint mobility.

Instructions

1. With neck in neutral position (neither flexed nor extended), cradle head in hands, while using the broad, soft pads of your fingers to palpate a single cervical vertebra's transverse processes.
2. Compare the left and right mobility of this single vertebra by translating (laterally moving) it along with the head and entire neck above your point of contact, without sidebending the neck.
3. When a translation restriction is found, gently but firmly press that vertebra in the more difficult direction using this vertebra as a fulcrum, and simultaneously sidebend the neck the opposite direction (direct technique). i.e., for difficulty translating left, press that vertebra left and sidebend the neck right.
4. Wait for softening or easing in the restricted direction. Repeat with each restricted vertebra. Alternatively, use reverse the direction of pressure for an indirect approach.
5. Variations: assess and release with cervicals in a slightly flexed or extended position, in addition to neutral position.

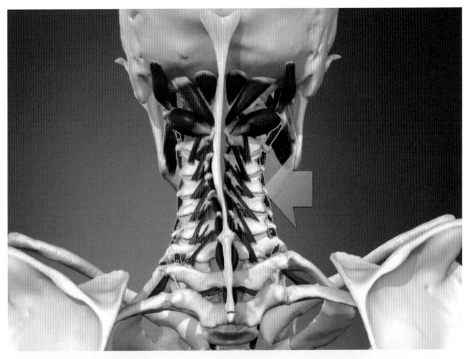

Figure 10.9

The ligamentous capsules of the facet joints (green) and the intertransverse ligaments and muscles (orange) are some of the structures that can limit translation. The arrow indicates placement and direction of pressure for a direct release of a vertebra that resists left translation.

Whole person, whole body

While the techniques presented in these two chapters will give you very effective tools for working with whiplash, it would be wrong to give the impression that they are all you'll need to be expert in this complex injury pattern.

Not only are the physical effects many, varied, and complex, but it is important to keep in mind that whiplash sufferers commonly experience body-mind effects such as persistent anxiety, depression, sleep disturbances, and many other biopsychosocial impacts (3). Even though direct treatment of these issues is outside the scope of most manual therapy practitioners, the psychosocial support that hands-on caregivers provide in the course of their normal work can be an important resource for clients dealing with whiplash injuries.

In spite of the complexity of whiplash injuries, myofascial techniques, when performed with skill and sensitivity, can be a very important part of whiplash recovery. Our faculty and alumni have numerous anecdotes from our own clinical experience; additionally, the effectiveness of a myofascial approach for improving neck function after whiplash has been demonstrated in at least one randomized controlled trial as well (4).

Most importantly, working with whiplash requires that the body is viewed as a whole. Whiplash is often a whole-body injury, and it is common to see pain or signs of injury anywhere. Many techniques for working the neck's superficial fascia and the deep posterior compartment described in the previous chapters will also be helpful for addressing both the autonomic aspect of hot whiplash, and the structural effects of cold whiplash.

Dr. Ida Rolf reportedly asked one of her structural integration classes: "Where in the body do you start working with whiplash?" Her students gave several well-reasoned answers—the sacrum, the jaw, the arms, the lower back. "Wrong," she said, "you start working whiplash at the big toe." (5) The implications of this point of view have inspired several generations of Rolfers and other integrative practitioners to study the complex interconnections that make up a living body.

Just as Advanced-Trainings.com faculty members Larry Koliha and George Sullivan write in the tips that follow, all of us can learn from Dr. Rolf's insight that whiplash is an entire-body phenomenon. As a result, untangling the effects of whiplash often means focusing less on the local injuries involved and more on the whole body—from the big toe up.

Strategizing your Sessions: Whiplash Tips from the Advanced Myofascial Techniques Faculty

Three of our lead instructors at Advanced-Trainings.com share some of their key considerations for strategizing whiplash sessions:

Tip 1. Prepare: Begin with light touch in the first session.

The trauma of whiplash and its after-effects can trigger hyper-arousal of the nervous system, which can make working with whiplash clients challenging. In hot whiplash, the nervous system of an injured person is in overload, and needs to be approached with care. Work gently to gauge how the client will respond, especially in the first session. Remain patient, and avoid aggravating the tissues and nervous system. Trying to get too much done in any one session can be overwhelming for the client. Even in cold whiplash, if you work too deeply too quickly, it can create more guarding and trauma.

Ellyn Vandenberg, Certified in Advanced Myofascial Techniques, Certified Rolfer

Tip 2. Differentiate: Work from appendicular to axial.

Imagine that you are sitting at a stop sign looking in your rearview mirror and you see the car behind you isn't slowing down and is about to hit you. You brace for impact by clutching the steering wheel and stomping both feet into the pedals and floor. This reaction is initiated to help protect the body from the impact that is about to occur. As a practitioner, if your client's arms and shoulder girdle are still compressed from this response, you cannot effectively release the neck. The same goes for the feet, legs, and pelvic girdle. Release the shoulders, arms, feet, legs, pelvic girdle, and low back early in your whiplash work. Working in these areas helps to release the protective compression these parts exert on the axial spine.

Larry Koliha, Certified in Advanced Myofascial Techniques, Certified Advanced Rolfer

Tip 3. Integrate: Be sure to integrate and close your work.

After working with whiplash, it is important to finish your session judiciously, making sure that primary shock points where injury can accumulate are left free and adaptable. The atlanto-occipital (A/O) junction is one of these places, and the therapeutic effects that cascade throughout the body by releasing restrictions at this neural/myofascial crossroads are difficult to overestimate. The sacroiliac (SI) joint is another; decompression of the myofascia here enables better adaptability and function at this critical structure. Working the SI joint complements and completes the circle of integration whenever having worked with the spine, neck, or upper body.

George Sullivan, Certified in Advanced Myofascial Techniques, Certified Advanced Rolfer

References

[1] Conlin, A., Bhogal, S., Sequeira, K. et al. (2005) Treatment of whiplash associated disorders – part I: Noninvasive interventions. *Pain Research & Management.* 10. p. 21–32.

[2] Bogduk, N. (2011) On cervical zygapophysial joint pain after whiplash. *Spine.* (Phila Pa 1976). Dec 1; 36(25 Suppl): S194–199.

[3] Gross, A.R., Kaplan, F., Huang, S., Khan, M., Santaguida, P.L., Carlesso, L.C. et al. (2013) Psychological care, patient education, orthotics, ergonomics and prevention strategies for neck pain: A systematic overview update as part of the ICON Project. *The Open Orthopaedics Journal.* 7. p. 530–561.

[4] Picelli, A., Ledro, G., Turrina, A., Stecco, C., Santilli, V., and Smania, N. (2011) Effects of myofascial technique in patients with subacute whiplash associated disorders: A pilot study. *European Journal of Physical and Rehabilitation Medicine.* 47(4). p. 561–568.

[5] This story was related to the author by William "Dub" Leigh, a manual therapist and student of Ida Rolf, during a training in 1985.

Picture credits

Study Guide

Cold Whiplash

1 Why does the chapter recommend against using lubricant in the initial stages of the Cervical Core/Sleeve Technique?

a to work deeper layers
b to avoid creating inflammation
c to avoid working too deep
d to better differentiate layers

2 Which active movement is recommended in the text for the Cervical Core/Sleeve technique?

a cervical rotation
b cervical sidebending
c cervical extension
d cervical flexion

3 What is the suggested method for releasing protective appendicular compression after a whiplash injury?

a work from appendicular to axial
b between the spinous processes
c work the atlanto-occipital (A/O) junction
d work the sacroiliac (SI) joint

4 When cervical translation is difficult to the client's right, in a direct approach, the text suggests pressure (a "fulcrum") on the immobile vertebra, and sidebending the neck:

a right
b left
c the easier direction
d the direction is not specified

5 Which cold whiplash goal is the Lateral Cervical Translation Technique primarily addressing?

a increase motility
b increase mobility
c calm ANS responses
d fascial layer differentiation

For Answer Keys, visit www.Advanced-Trainings.com/v2key/

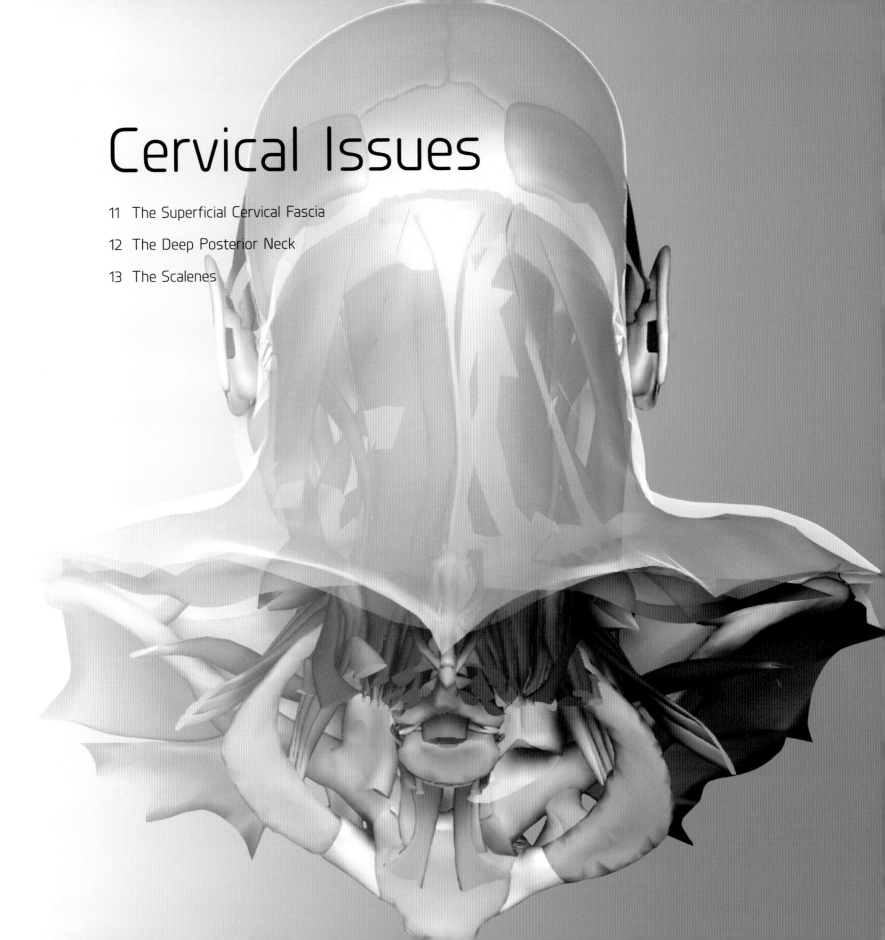

Cervical Issues

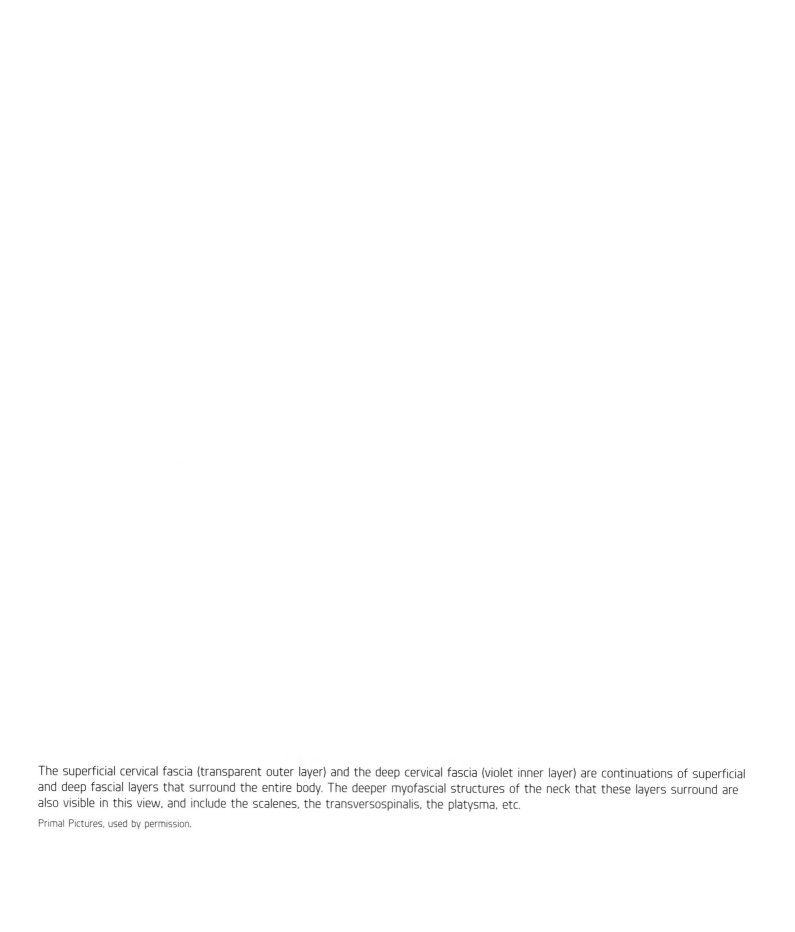

The superficial cervical fascia (transparent outer layer) and the deep cervical fascia (violet inner layer) are continuations of superficial and deep fascial layers that surround the entire body. The deeper myofascial structures of the neck that these layers surround are also visible in this view, and include the scalenes, the transversospinalis, the platysma, etc.

The Superficial Cervical Fascia

The Importance of the Superficial Layers

What are the most common client issues that you see in your practice? Chances are, neck pain and discomfort are high on the list. Although cervical complaints and conditions can have many causes, you'll almost always see better results if you begin your work with these very common issues by addressing restrictions in the superficial layers of the neck and shoulders. Whether caused by deep articular fixations, posture and misalignment, habits, stress, injury, or other reasons, neck issues respond quicker and stay away longer when the differentiation and elasticity of the outer wrappings is addressed first. As with other parts of the body, many seemingly deeper neck issues resolve when the external layers have been freed. In this chapter, I'll describe how to work with these superficial but important layers, which will also prepare for working the neck's deeper structures (which are covered in the next chapter).

Encircling the neck and shoulders like an over-large turtleneck sweater, or a surgical collar (Figures 11.1 and 11.2), the neck's outer wrappings are composed of multiple layers of myofascia. These include superficial layers just under the skin (such as the fascia colli in back, and the fascia colli superficialis in front), as well as the investing fascia that surrounds the outer neck muscles (such as the trapezius, sternocleidomastoid, infrahyoids, and the platysma, Figure 11.3). Together, these cowl-like superficial layers extend from their superior attachments on the occipital ridge and convergence with the fascia of the lower face, to their merging with the outer layers of the shoulders, chest, and upper back at their inferior margin (1). Like a sleeve, they

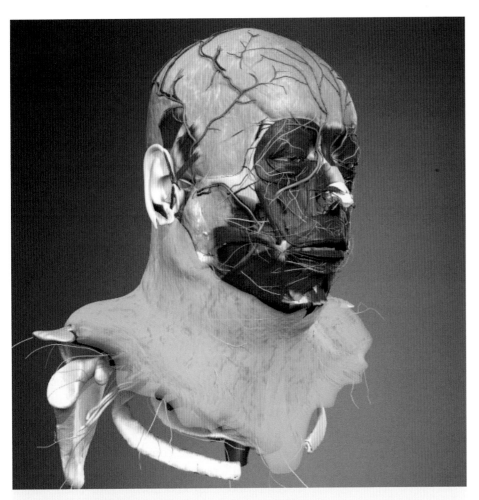

Figures 11.1/11.2 (overleaf)

The superficial fascia of the neck, in green, surrounds the deeper cervical structures, like a sleeve or cowl. It is continuous with similar layers in the face, head, shoulders, back, and chest.

109

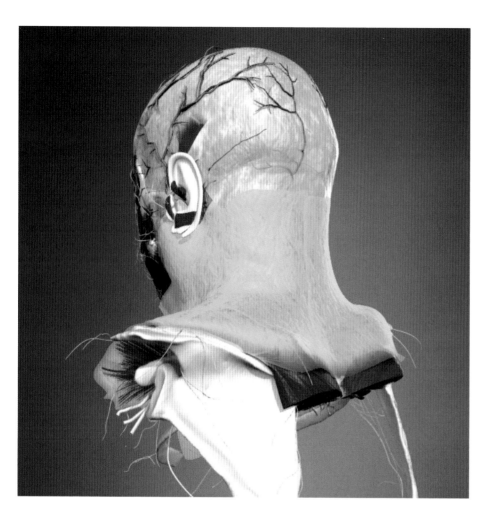

encircle the deeper myofascial, skeletal, and visceral structures of the neck's core.

The outer layers of the neck have a surprising thickness and resilience. When they lose pliability or are undifferentiated and adhered to other structures (due to injury, postural strain, or other reasons), the outer layers have the ability to restrict movement range, disrupt balanced alignment, and bind the structures they surround. Imagine trying to move in a wetsuit that is a size too small (Figure 11.4)—the outer layers of the neck can tether, distort, and constrain movement in the same way. And the thickness, elasticity, and sliding of these layers can directly correlate to pain. In one ultrasound study of living subjects, neck pain was seen to be proportional to the thickness of the cervical fasciae, which in turn was observed to measurably change as a result of hands-on fascial techniques (2). In another ultrasound study, sliding between fascial layers in people with neck or back pain has been seen to measurably improve after myofascial work (3).

Assessing superficial restrictions

Try this: observe your standing client turn his or her head from side to side. Watch what happens with the superficial layers of the neck, shoulders, chest, and back. Are there areas of the torso's fascia that move along with the head and neck? Or, do you see lines of tension and pull appearing in the skin and outer layers? Often, these signs of fascial inelasticity, binding, and lack of differentiation will be most visible at the extremes or end-range of the movement. Look from both the front and the back; compare left and right sides for any differences. Then, look again as he or she gently looks up and down. Your client might feel different kinds of restrictions when moving; including pulls in the deeper musculature, or catches involving neck articulations or the

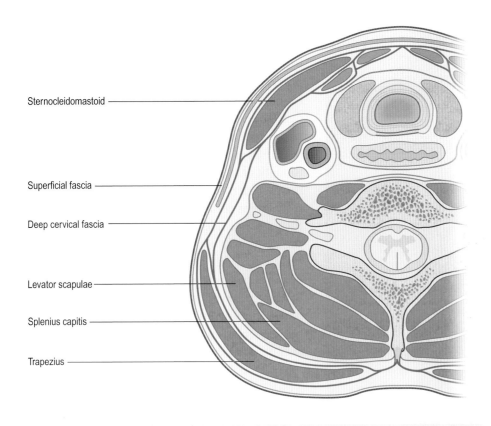

Sternocleidomastoid

Superficial fascia

Deep cervical fascia

Levator scapulae

Splenius capitis

Trapezius

Figure 11.3

The superficial layers of the neck, in cross-section (after an illustration from Ida Rolf's 1979 "The Integration of Human Structures").

upper ribs. For now, we're going to leave these aside and focus on the outer layers first.

Sometimes superficial fascial tension will be visible as linear "tug" patterns in the skin (Figure 11.5). In other cases, a whole sheet of fascia will move or creep along with the rotating or nodding head. Linear "tug" patterns are more commonly seen in the thinner layers of the anterior neck and chest, while the "creep" of whole fascial sheets is seen more often when looking at the thicker posterior layers of the back.

If it is difficult to see restrictions in the superficial layers, you can use your hands instead to feel for tugs and pulls in the outer layers while your client rotates his or her head. Whether watching or feeling, note any areas that don't display a smooth, even lengthening of the dermis and superficial fasciae when the head moves.

When testing for fascial tension with active movement, don't confuse movements of deeper structures for movement in the superficial fascia. For example, you'll sometimes see the ribcage turning along with the head, or a shoulder roll forward, etc. Some of this movement is normal; if you see exaggerated or asymmetrical movement of the ribcage or shoulder, this might be because of deeper or larger restrictions. Make a note to check for and address these patterns later, but remember that since these deeper movements might also be caused by restrictions in the outer layers, releasing the superficial layers is the logical first step.

Releasing Superficial Restrictions

Once you've seen or felt where your client's outer layers are tugging or creeping along with head and neck movement, you can go to work. A word about sequencing your superficial work on the upper torso: most clients will feel more balanced if you begin by working the posterior restrictions

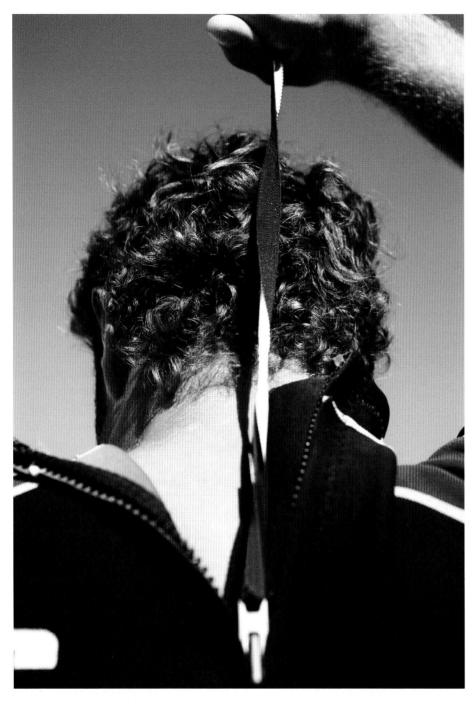

Figure 11.4
The superficial layers of the neck can restrict motion of the neck, jaw, shoulders and chest, much like a too-tight wetsuit might.

of the upper back, and end by addressing the anterior restrictions. This is the order we're using in this chapter. Why this back-to-front progression? Since most of us tend to have our heads forward of the coronal midline to some degree, and are narrower across the front of our chest than across our upper back, the anterior fascial layers of the chest and shoulders can be thought of as shorter than the posterior layers of the shoulders and back. Ending with the anterior restrictions counterbalances the earlier work on the posterior side of the body, and usually leaves the client with a greater sense of anterior width, length, and freedom, and so helps with overall postural balance and ease. A possible exception to this ordering: if your client has a very flat upper thoracic curve, you may want to reverse the sequence, and end with work on the back to encourage more spinal flexion.

Over-The-Edge Technique

Ask your client to lie face down on your table, arms at the sides, with his or her head and neck just over the top edge of the table. The edge of the table should fall an inch or two below the top of the sternum. Your client may need to adjust upwards or downwards a bit so that the edge is comfortable. You won't want to leave your client like this too long, but you'll usually have at least two or three minutes to work before his or her head starts to feel too full.

Once your client is comfortable, ask for active side-to-side head and neck rotation, as you observe again or feel the outer tissue layers. This allows you to recheck your findings, and compare this pattern to what you saw in an upright stance. Look at the flexion/extension (up-and-down) movements too, again using care to avoid excessive neck compression with extension. Because the effects of gravity are different in this position, you may see or feel additional

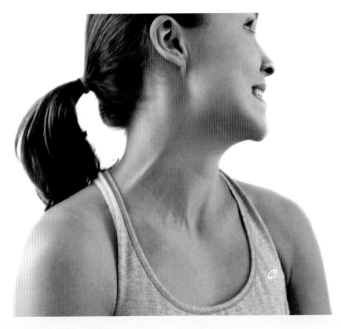

Figure 11.5
Assessing superficial restrictions: fascial strain visible as "tugging" of the outer layers with head rotation.

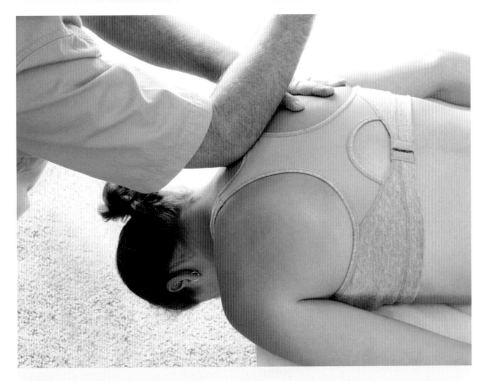

Figure 11.6
The Over-the-Edge Technique for addressing the superficial layers of the upper back and shoulders. Although relatively safe, head-down positions are usually contraindicated for clients with uncontrolled high blood pressure, glaucoma, a history or risk of strokes, vertigo, or acute sinus issues.

undifferentiated areas that weren't obvious in standing. Often, this prone position will make the superficial restrictions even more obvious.

The tool we'll use to differentiate these less-pliable layers is the flat of our forearm; specifically, the first few inches of the ulna just distal to the elbow (Figure 11.6). Use this tool to gently anchor the inferior margins of the areas where you saw or felt superficial restrictions. Don't use oil or cream; we'll be using friction more than pressure to contact the layer we want to release. Also, we won't be sliding much—different from a passive "stroke," our client will actively provide the movement needed for layer differentiation and increasing elasticity.

Once you have the outer layers gently but firmly anchored with your forearm, ask your client to slowly turn his or her head away from the side you're working. Feel for the direction of your pressure that gently lengthens the superficial layers being pulled on by the head movement. Imagine that you're helping your client lengthen and free herself inside the wetsuit-like outer layers of superficial fascia.

Alternatively, you can ask your client to lift and lower the head (extend and flex the neck and spine) as you lengthen the layers of the back inferiorly. You'll find this technique most effective on the eccentric phase of the motion, that is, while your client is lowering his or her head.

Remember, your client may become uncomfortable if you leave them in this position for more than a few minutes. Although relatively safe, head-down positions are probably contraindicated for clients with uncontrolled high blood pressure, glaucoma, history or risk of strokes, vertigo, or acute sinus issues.

See video of the Over-the-Edge Technique at www.a-t.tv/wb08

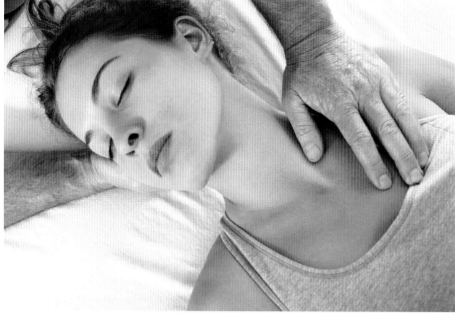

Figure 11.7
An open palm or the tips of curled fingers may be used to anchor the pectoralis fascia in the Cervical/Pectoralis Fascia Technique.

Key points: Over-the-Edge Technique

Indications include:
- Neck, shoulder, or back pain.
- Movement restrictions or stiffness.
- Fascial layer creep or tug observed with neck rotation.

Purpose
- Increase fascial layer differentiation, elasticity, and gliding.
- Prepare the neck and shoulders for deeper work.

Instructions
1. Position prone client with head and neck comfortably off the end of the table; the edge of the table should be just below the collarbone.
2. Use the broad, flat section of your ulna, just distal to the elbow, to anchor layers caudally. Ask for active client movement.

Movements
- Active rotation, nodding, and/or sidebending of the neck.

Precautions
- Avoid uncomfortable hyperextension of the neck – cue client to keep neck long while lifting the head.
- Contraindicated for clients with uncontrolled high blood pressure; glaucoma; history or risk of stroke; vertigo; acute or unstable neck injuries (including hot whiplash); or acute sinus issues.
- Monitor client's comfort, and limit time in this position to two to three minutes maximum.

Cervical/Pectoralis Fascia Technique

After differentiating the superficial layers of the back and posterior shoulders, broaden and continue this release by addressing any surface restrictions in the upper chest and anterior shoulders.

To release these anterior restrictions, use either palms or fingertips to gently anchor the superficial fascia of the shoulders, chest, and anterior

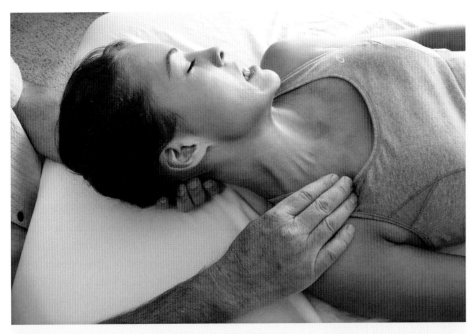

Figure 11.8
Active contraction of the platysma, as in grimacing, can aid in increasing elasticity and differentiation of the superficial fascia of the anterior neck and thorax.

neck (Figure 11.7). Then, use your client's active movements to release the restrictions you saw or felt earlier. The palm is especially useful where you saw fascial layers creep with head movement. When using your palm, don't be tempted yet to rub, slide, or massage the deeper layers of pectoralis muscle. Instead, use the broad surface of the palm to catch and gently anchor the outer layers of the chest, while your client moves his or her head.

In contrast to the broad tool of the palm, using the fingertips will allow you to work very specific areas, and so are useful where you saw local tugs in the outer layers. The fingers are slightly curved rather than straight, and can sensitively "hook in" to the outer layer you saw or felt moving with the head. Push with your fingertips, as if straightening out your curled fingers, to encourage superficial release away from the direction of movement.

Whether you're using palm or fingertips, don't slide along the surface, and don't dig down to the pectoral muscles, ribs, or intercostals—you want to feel a tug in the outer strata, the layers of dermis and superficial fascia that lie between the actual surface of the skin, and the muscles or bones beneath.

Movement: as in the Over-the-Edge Technique, ask your client to slowly turn the head away from the side you're anchoring. Find a direction for your pressure that gently releases the superficial layers being pulled by the head movement. Imagine that you're helping your client lengthen and free him or herself inside the wetsuit-like outer layers of superficial fascia.

A further option is to have your client tighten the platysma muscle, which lies within the superficial fasciae that you're working. Try it yourself as you're reading this—turn your head, and then grimace or snarl until you feel a tug from your lower lip into the pectoral fascia of your chest.

By using your hand to anchor the lower end of this tug in the chest, you can snarl and relax repeatedly in order to release any inelasticity

Key points: Cervical/Pectoralis Fascia Technique

Indications include:
- Neck, jaw, face, or shoulder pain.
- Movement restrictions of the neck, jaw, face, chest, or shoulders.
- TMJ pain or misalignment.
- Torticollis or postural issues.
- Fascial layer creep or tug observed with neck rotation, arm movement, or breathing.

Purpose
- Increase fascial layer differentiation, elasticity, and gliding.
- Prepare the neck, shoulders, face, or chest for deeper work.

Instructions
1. Use a broad palm to anchor the superficial fascia of the shoulders, chest, and anterior neck.
2. Use slightly curved finger tips to hook and work more specific areas.
3. Ask for slow active movement. Cue client to slow down further or stop and wait for release, whenever you feel fascial restrictions.

Movements
- Slow, active neck rotation.
- Active contraction of the platysma as in grimacing, frowning, or sneering, feeling for connection of these movements to areas of fascial inelasticity.

in the anterior cervical and pectoralis fasciae (Figure 11.8). Asking your client to tighten and relax the platysma in this way while you anchor its inferior attachments can help him or her focus the work into the most restricted areas.

Finishing

Once you've worked with the outer layers of the neck and torso from both the back and front, look again as your client turns his or her head from side to side. If you've been both patient and thorough, you'll see fewer pulls and tugs in the outer layers, and more than likely, smoother and greater range of motion. Clients often report that their movement feels easier, freer, or that their head is lighter and more upright.

Now that you've addressed the outer layers, the next step could be deeper work with the neck, ribcage, or spine, either in the same session, or during the next appointment. The deeper work will now be easier, more effective, and longer lasting. Or, instead of working deeper right away, you might want to continue the theme of superficial release first by adapting the techniques we've just done here to other regions of the body, such as the lumbars, limbs, or hips. You can find techniques for these areas in other chapters of these volumes. In the meantime, keep investigating what happens when you take time to release the outer layers of the body.

References

[1] Breul, R. (2012) The deeper fasciae of the neck and ventral torso. In: Robert Schleip et al. (eds). *Fascia: The Tensional Network of the Human Body.* Elsevier. p. 46.

[2] Stecco, A., Meneghini, A., Stern, R., Stecco, C., and Imamura, M. (2013) Ultrasonography in myofascial neck pain: Randomized clinical trial for diagnosis and follow-up. *Surgical and Radiologic Anatomy.* Aug 23.

[3] Tozzi, P., Bongiorno, D., and Vitturini, C. (2011) Fascial release effects on patients with non-specific cervical or lumbar pain. *Journal of Bodywork and Movement Therapies.* 15(4): 405–416.

Picture credits

Figures 11.1 and 11.2 courtesy Primal Pictures, used by permission.
Figure 11.3 courtesy estate of John Lodge, used by permission.
Figure 11.4 Thinkstock.
Figures 11.5 – 11.8 courtesy Advanced-Trainings.com.

Study Guide
The Superficial Cervical Fascia

1 **Where does the text say that linear skin "tug" patterns are most commonly seen when turning the head?**

a posterior neck
b posterior upper back
c anterior neck and chest
d anterior lower jaw

2 **What reason is given for ending the superficial work on the anterior body, vs. on the back?**

a Finishing this way leaves the client with a sense of strength, which is stabilizing for most people.
b Finishing this way leaves the client with a sense of width, which is balancing for most people.
c Finishing this way is how Ida Rolf did it.
d No reason is given for finishing with superficial work on the chest.

3 **The chapter recommends not keeping the client face down in the Over-the-Edge Technique for longer than:**

a 20 to 60 seconds
b two to three minutes
c three to six minutes
d two to three sessions

4 **What is the practitioner's ulna feeling for in the Over-the-Edge Technique?**

a fascial lengthening of the upper back
b fascial differentiation of the anterior neck
c fascial differentiation on the front of the body
d fascial differentiation of the lower jaw

5 **What client movement is mentioned for the Cervical/Pectoralis Fascia Technique?**

a pelvic tilt
b arm rotation
c lifting the eyebrows
d snarl or grimace

For Answer Keys, visit www.Advanced-Trainings.com/v2key/

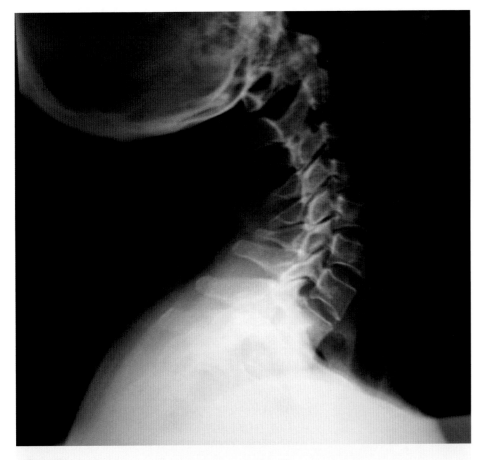

Figure 12.1
Cervical hyperextension.

Whether addressing stubborn neck pain, postural issues, or cold whiplash (Chapter 10), working with the deepest structures in the neck will often yield results that nothing else can. In the previous chapter, *The Superficial Cervical Fascia*, I mentioned how taking time to release superficial restrictions before working deeper structures, can increase your effectiveness and give longer-lasting results. In this chapter, we'll look at ways to assess and release deeper neck restrictions. Since this is essentially Part II of the previous chapter, I'll assume you've done some work to release and prepare the superficial fascial layers before attempting the techniques here.

The Nod Test

See video of the
Nod Test at
www.a-t.tv/nb02

The Nod Test allows us to assess three important things:

1. Freedom at the atlanto-occipital (A/O) joint;
2. The ability of the posterior compartment of the neck to lengthen; and
3. The degree of participation of the "prevertebral" muscles along the front of the cervical spine.

Each of these contribute to the alignment, flexibility, and stability of the neck, particularly when working with "head forward" positions (cervical lordosis, or chronic hyperextension, Figure 12.1).[1]

Begin with your client sitting or standing. While looking at his or her profile, ask for small nodding motions. We want just a little bit of movement—too much will make the initiation of movement hard to see. As you watch these small movements, ask yourself:

- Which neck joint moves first?
- Which joint or joints are not flexing and extending?

1 In my experience, the most common challenges to neck alignment involve shortened structures in the posterior neck, and relative lack of engagement of the deep prevertebral muscles in front. Together, these cause the neck to rest in an extended, "head forward," or lordotic position. In the opposite pattern, such as the true "military neck," there is diminished cervical extension and a straighter neck. Although "military neck" is a common diagnosis, in my experience, problems arising from a hyper-erect neck are less common than those connected to lordotic neck patterns, so working with a lordotic pattern is emphasized in this chapter.

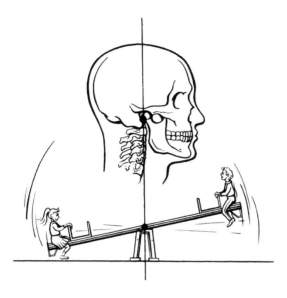

Figure 12.2

When the soft-tissue structures around the atlanto-occipital joint are free, small nodding motions will happen primarily at the top of the neck, allowing the occiput to balance and move on the atlas like a seesaw.

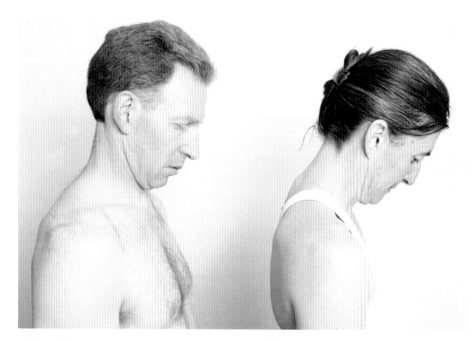

Figure 12.3

The Nod Test. When the deep structures of the posterior neck are able to lengthen in the larger motions of cervical flexion, nodding happens primarily at the top of the neck (as on the left). When the posterior compartment cannot lengthen, cervical flexion is limited, and the motion of nodding gets driven into the base of the neck (as on the right).

If it is hard to see these things, ask your client to make even smaller motions, while you look for the very first joints that move, and for joints that don't move. You can also use your hands to feel for this initiation, if it still isn't clear through visual assessment.

This simple small-nodding test helps you find both where most of your client's cervical flexion and extension typically occurs, and where it is not moving. By implication, you can determine if there is freedom at the topmost joint of the neck, the atlanto-occipital joint (A/O). When the soft-tissue structures around the A/O are free, small nodding motions will primarily happen here, allowing the head to balance and rock on the atlas like a seesaw (Figure 12.2). When it is present, this top-of-the-neck freedom gives a sense of lightness and poise. If the motion appears to be happening lower in the neck instead of at the A/O, it could indicate restrictions in the suboccipital or transversospinalis myofascia.

Once you've assessed A/O freedom with small motions, ask your client to do larger nodding, as in looking up and down (Figure 12.3). With this larger motion, look for the ability of the posterior compartment of the neck to lengthen in flexion. One way to see this is to look for evenness of flexion and extension throughout the cervical column. When the posterior structures can't lengthen, larger nodding motions are driven lower in the neck, and the middle and upper cervical joints typically have less flexion.

Transversospinalis Technique

In a client who has limited neck flexion, as in the person on the right in Figure 12.3, the Transversospinalis Technique is an effective way to increase the elasticity and differentiation of the strong, middle-level longitudinal structures, including the outer splenius and trapezius, the

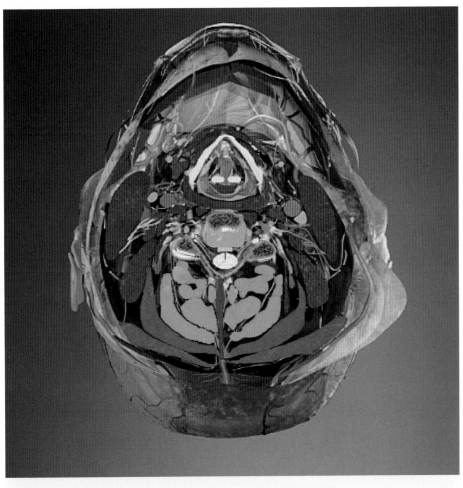

Figure 12.4

Cross-section of the neck at C5, from below. Shortened soft-tissue structures of the posterior neck, here colored green, can contribute to limited flexion and increased cervical lordosis. These structures include the outer splenius and trapezius (medium green), the central nuchal ligament (dark green), and the deeper transversospinalis group (bright green).

central nuchal ligament, and the deeper transversospinalis group (Figure 12.4).

We'll use the first knuckles (the proximal interphalangeal or PIP joints) to anchor and lengthen these deep layers (Figure 12.5). Seated comfortably at the client's head, place your right forearm and wrist on the table for stability. With the PIP knuckles of your first two fingers, gently feel for longitudinal shortness in the various layers of the deeper neck structures, first on the right side of the neck. Anchor these short tissues in a caudal or foot-ward direction.

Once you've comfortably placed your right hand, you can slowly bring your client's neck into a bit of flexion. With the left forearm braced against the edge of the table for stability, lift the head to slightly flex the neck. When you get your position and angles right, lifting the head is relatively easy, even if your client is bigger than you. If lifting the head feels like a strain, reposition until you find an easier way. Even though your right hand is stationary on the table, lifting the head has the effect of dragging the tissues out from under your knuckles. Keep your pace slow and steady, feeling for restrictions in the posterior compartment of the neck, and wait, rather than push, for release.

Once you've made an initial pass or two, you can focus on very detailed work into particularly tight or short structures by incrementally lifting, rotating, flexing, and extending the neck around the point of contact, all the while encouraging length up the back of the neck. Be thorough, working deeper through the various layers you encounter, all the way from the occipital ridge into the shoulders and base of the neck. By switching your hand position, you can work the left and right, as well as the central nuchal ligament (taking care not to apply an uncomfortable level of pressure directly to the spinous processes).

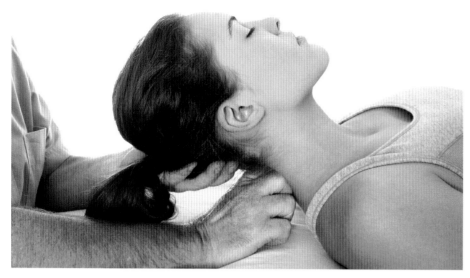

Figure 12.5

In the Transversospinalis Technique, you'll slowly lift the client's head while gently anchoring shortened structures of the posterior neck. The knuckles provide a strong, sensitive, and stable tool. Be sure to keep your wrist as straight as possible.

Key points: Transversospinalis Technique

Indications include:
- Lack of posterior cervical compartment lengthening with large flexion motions of the Nod Test.
- Head-forward posture and cervical lordosis.
- Immobility related to cold whiplash (Chapter 10).
- Tension and myofascial headaches (Chapter 16).

Purpose
- Increase evenness of cervical flexion by lengthening the neck's posterior compartment.

Instructions

While your left hand supports and lifts your supine client's head into flexion:

1. Use your first knuckles (PIP joints) of your right hand to anchor the tissues alongside the cervical spine, stabilizing your arm with the edge of the table.
2. Slowly lift the head (flex the neck) to lengthen tissues caudally by dragging them past your static right hand.
3. Work both the right and left sides of the posterior neck, as well as gently on the center nuchal ligament (avoiding uncomfortable pressure on the spinous processes).

Cervical Wedge Technique

It is one thing to release restricted tissues, and it is another to help our clients find new ways of moving that will prevent the restrictions from returning. This technique can do both— it is an effective way to release deep soft-tissue restrictions, right down to the deepest articulations of the cervical spinal column; and in the active-motion version, it will help your client find new movement possibilities that will support the structural work once the session is over.

Use the fingertips of both hands to feel the space and tissue texture beside and between the spinous processes of two vertebrae; begin at the base of the neck with C6 and C7. Work head-ward, checking each articulation that you can palpate. Gently lift with your fingertips into any restricted spaces

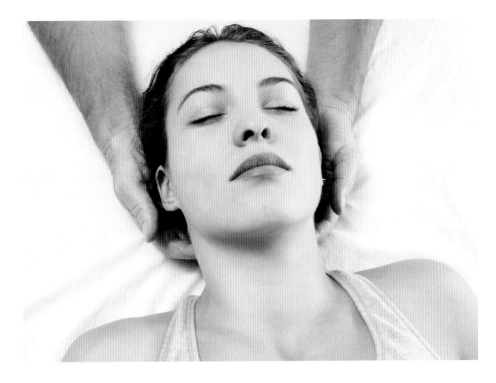

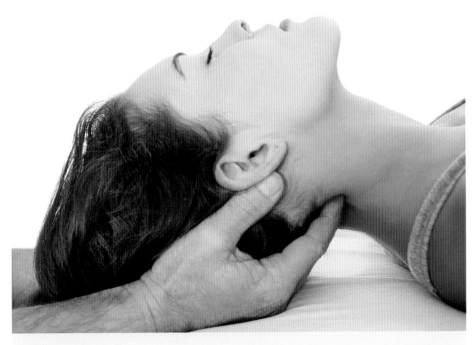

Figures 12.6/12.7

In the Cervical Wedge Technique, use the fingertips of both hands to feel beside and between the spinous processes of each neck vertebra for any crowded or immobile spaces. Wait for each joint to open in response to your pressure, rather than trying to "drive" the wedge of your fingers in. Use guided active movement to refine proprioceptive awareness of flexion and extension.

between the spinous processes (Figure 12.6 and 12.7). Keep your hands relaxed onto the table to avoid straining; lift with just the fingertips.

When the neck flexes, the space between these cervical spinous processes opens. In a neck that has lost flexion, like the one shown on the right in Figure 12.3 (the Nod Test), some of the spaces between the spinous processes will be crowded and tight (most often between the 3rd and 4th cervical vertebrae). Your fingertips are the wedges that can help invite more space at each joint. However, don't drive the wedge in, as if splitting a piece of firewood. Rather than forcing the joint open, let your finger pressure be like a flashlight, showing your client where new space and length is possible. At each tight space, wait for the client's tissues and nervous system to respond to your touch. Be sure to spend time at the top joint of the neck, the A/O, especially if your small-nodding test showed movement restriction here.

In the passive version of this technique, simply find the shortened spaces between the spinous processes of the neck with your fingertips, and in each place, wait for the cervical joints to open around the wedge of your fingertips. In the active variation, once you find a shortened space between two cervical vertebrae, ask for small, subtle nodding motions. Coach your client until you both feel the first movement of nodding occurring right at the joint space in question. In addition to releasing shortened tissues, your client gains proprioceptive access to the joints that weren't opening as much as others.

At first it may be difficult for your client to focus their nodding motion at the articulations that aren't accustomed to moving. Some of the verbal cues you can use include:

- "Use very small movements to let this space open."
- "Leave your head heavy on the table. Let the movement begin right here."
- "Let the back of your head move upward on the table to gently open this space."

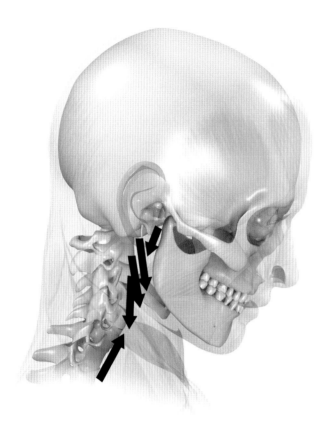

Figure 12.8

The active version of the Cervical Wedge Technique engages the prevertebral muscles along the front of the spine (arrows) to help open any narrowed spaces between posterior spinous processes. In a hyper-erect or "military neck" pattern, the wedge technique can be reversed to encourage more extension (posterior closing) between cervical vertebrae.

You may need to start with other joints, where there is already obvious flexion and extension with nodding; once you and your client can both feel the motion at a mobile articulation, you can move up or down into the more restricted joints.

Another pointer: often, practitioners and clients start with movements that are too large to allow the specificity required. We're teaching the ability to initiate flexion and extension at specific cervical joints, and this almost always involves asking our clients to slow down, and to make even smaller movements than they're accustomed to. Be patient, stay in conversation with your client, and encourage him or her whenever you feel movement at the restricted joint. Although subtle, the movement will be clear and tangible to both of you when you've established it.

Incidentally, the back-of-the-neck lengthening that we're looking for involves more than just releasing the posterior joint spaces—it also involves engaging the *prevertebral muscles* along the anterior side of the spine: the longus capitis, rectus capitis anterior, and longus colli (Figure 12.8). These deep front-side antagonists to the posterior neck extensors help balance and coordinate cervical flexion and extension. In a cervical lordosis pattern, they are typically under-utilized. The active version of the "wedge" technique automatically engages these prevertebral muscles; you'll be increasing their participation in movement and posture when you're helping your client find flexion at each restricted joint.

In a hyper-erect or "military neck" pattern, use the active wedge technique in reverse i.e. encourage more extension (posterior closing) between cervical vertebrae. Find the most open or flexed vertebral spaces. Then, as you use your wedge to indicate these places to your client, coach him or her to gently pinch or close right around your fingers. Go for subtlety, specificity, and the ability to initiate extension right at the joint in question. Of course, it is important to avoid over-extending the neck, so stay focused on local extension at specific joints.

Key points: Cervical Wedge Technique

Indications include:
- Lack of cervical and suboccipital flexion with small and large movements of the Nod Test.
- Head-forward posture and cervical lordosis.
- Flat or reversed cervical curves ("military neck").
- Immobility related to cold whiplash (Chapter 10).
- Tension and myofascial headaches (Chapter 16).

Purpose
- Increase mobility, participation, proprioception of all cervical joints in flexion and extension.
- Increase participation of prevertebral (anterior neck) muscles in flexion.

Instructions
1. Visually or tactilely identify any cervical joints with restricted flexion or extension using the Nod Test.
2. Lift with fingertips into the space between two immobile vertebrae to increase client's proprioceptive awareness.
3. Wait for the tissues to yield, then cue exploratory active movements.

Movements
- Encourage small, exploratory movements, guiding your client to initiate slight neck flexion at immobile joints, opening each joint at your fingertips.
- With "military neck" patterns, reverse the movement by guiding your client to initiate slight neck extension at immobile joints, closing each joint around your fingertips.

Remember the big picture

These techniques are quite effective, and you'll see satisfying results by using them. Of course, lasting change in neck patterns often involves more than just freeing local restrictions. More than just about anywhere else, the neck reflects support or mobility issues in the rest of the body. Issues such as eye strain (1), jaw issues (2), (3), shoulder pain (4), upper rib or pleural restrictions (5), vertebral immobility (Chapter 1), hip or pelvis asymmetries, or even support issues involving the lower limbs, can conceivably cause or reinforce neck posture and mobility issues. Other neck structures, particularly the scalenes (Chapter 13, *The Scalenes*) and sternocleidomastoids will be important to address as well.

Habits of posture and body use can be slow to change. So, don't be discouraged if you find neck issues that don't seem to respond initially. Think larger; learn more; refer to a Rolfer or other complementary practitioner who specializes in big-picture, integrative work, or in movement and posture re-education. And don't be afraid to experiment with these ideas and techniques and make them your own—your clients will undoubtedly benefit and your own level of satisfaction will increase.

References

[1] Mohandoss, M. et al. (2014) Comorbidities of myofascial neck pain among Information Technology professionals. *Annals of Occupational and Environmental Medicine.* 26(21). http://www.aoemj.com/content/26/1/21. [Accessed December 2015]

[2] Matheus, R.A. et al. (2009) The relationship between temporomandibular dysfunction and head and cervical posture. *Journal of Applied Oral Science.* 17(3). p. 204–208.

[3] Walczyńska-Dragon, K. et al. (2014) Correlation between TMD and cervical spine pain and mobility: Is the whole body balance TMJ related? *BioMed Research International.* Article ID 582414, 7 pages. http://doi:10.1155/2014/582414 [Accessed August 2015]

[4] Mohandoss, M. (2014) ibid.

[5] Charalampidis, C. et al. Pleura space anatomy. *Journal of Thoracic Disease* 7. Suppl 1: S27–S32. PMC.

Picture credits

12.1 Thinkstock.

Figure 12.2 courtesy Eric Franklin, originator of the Franklin Method (www.franklin-method.com), from his book *Dynamic Alignment through Imagery*, used by permission.

Figures 12.3, 12.5, 12.6, and 12.7 Advanced-Trainings.com

12.4 courtesy of Primal Pictures, used by permission.

Figure 12.8 from Kapandji, *Physiology of the Joints*, Volume III. All rights owned by Elsevier, Inc., used by permission.

Study Guide

The Deep Posterior Neck

1 **According to the text, when the soft tissue is free, the small movements of the Nod Test happen primarily at which joint(s)?**

a atlanto-occipital (A/O) joint
b C2–C3
c C7–T1
d all cervical joints equally

2 **What does the practitioner look for in the large movements of the Nod Test?**

a lengthening of the anterior neck
b lengthening of the posterior neck
c see-saw motion at the A/O joint
d lengthening in the lateral neck

3 **Where does the practitioner place their fingers in the Posterior Wedge Technique?**

a on the spinous processes
b between the spinous processes
c on the transverse processes
d between the transverse processes

4 **As mentioned in the text, which muscles are engaged in the active version of the Posterior Wedge Technique?**

a suboccipital extensors
b cervical extensors
c prevertebral flexors
d trapezius and levator scapula

5 **What active cervical movement is suggested for working with a hyper-erect or "military neck" in the Posterior Wedge Technique?**

a extension
b flexion
c rotation
d sidebending

For Answer Keys, visit www.Advanced-Trainings.com/v2key/

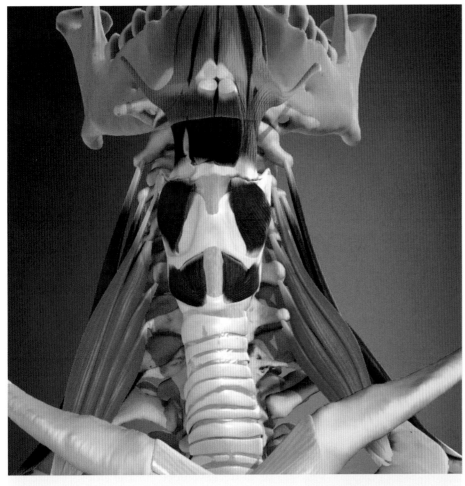

Figure 13.1

The scalenes' angled orientation enables them to play an integral part in numerous neck, arm, and rib conditions. In this image, the anterior scalenes are green, and the medial and posterior scalenes are red. (Also in red are the muscles of the floor of the mouth and anterior larynx.)

It is the scalenes' slanting, inclined, and tilted orientation that gives them their name. "Scalene" is a transliteration of the Greek σκαληνός, meaning "skew": neither parallel nor perpendicular (1). This angled arrangement of these deep cervical structures (Figure 13.1), in addition to making the scalenes powerful side-benders and rotators of the neck, puts them in position to align and stabilize the upright cervical column, much like the angled rigging of an ship's mast. (Figure 13.2).

At least, that's how the scalenes function when they're balanced. When they're shorter or tighter on one side, their angled left/right and anterior/posterior arrangement can cause them to literally "skew" the neck and upper ribs. This means that the scalenes are involved in numerous postural and positional issues, such as:

- Torticollis (wry neck) is a persistent and often-painful torsion of the neck, typically accompanied by asymmetrical scalene spasm and rigidity (2).
- In both head-forward postures as well as the "dowager's hump" pattern, the anterior scalenes are often hard, tight, and short, pulling the lower cervical vertebrae forward into a rigidly flexed position (Figure 13.3) (3).
- Although usually considered cervical flexors, once the neck is extended (as in the cervical lordosis that often accompanies a head-forward position), the anterior scalenes can become cervical extensors. This change in function is a result of their upper and lower attachments now both being posterior to the articulations they affect, making it impossible for the scalenes to counterbalance the lack of length in

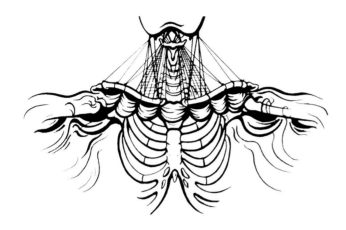

Figure 13.2

The soft tissue and bones of the neck, compared to a ship's angled rigging and upright mast.

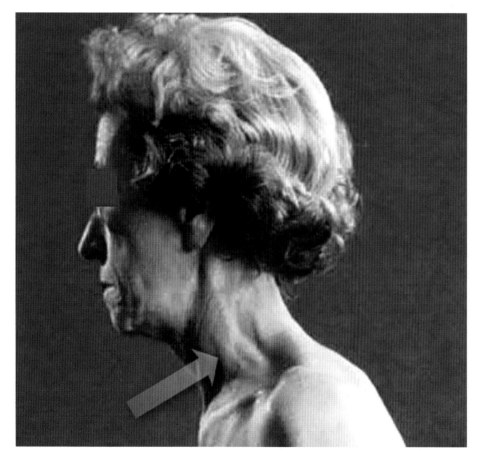

Figure 13.3

In head-forward postures, the scalenes (arrow) are often contracted and inelastic.

the posterior neck (Figure 13.4). Shortness in the scalenes will thus perpetuate and reinforce a cervical lordosis.

The scalenes are involved in other conditions as well:

- The scalenes are often injured in whiplash injuries, especially when lateral forces are involved. (Although working the scalenes can dramatically aid recovery from whiplash, this work is most appropriate with "cold" whiplash—fixed, chronic, older injuries. Direct work on the scalenes can aggravate whiplash symptoms when applied too soon after an injury; too aggressively; or in the presence of "hot" whiplash signs—muscular spasm, autonomic activation, instability, or guarding. (For more about hot and cold whiplash, see Chapters 9 and 10.)

- Because the scalenes also aid in forced inspiration by lifting the first two ribs, they are often chronically shortened when there are respiratory issues, such as emphysema or asthma.

- The scalenes stabilize the base of the neck against the asymmetrical forces of being right- or left-handed. For this reason, in people who habitually use their dominant hand to apply force (such as manual therapists), the scalenes are often significantly tighter or more developed on the side opposite the dominant hand.

- The deep pleural ligaments (Figure 13.5: transversopleural, vertebropleural, and, not pictured, costopleural) are fibrous bands that anchor the endothoracic fascia around the lungs to C7, T1, and the first rib. Lying deep to the scalenes and roughly parallel to their oblique arrangement, the pleural ligaments can have effects similar to the scalenes on the alignment and mobility of the base of the neck. (4)

Because the nerves of the brachial plexus pass between the anterior and the medial scalenes, crowding here can exacerbate symptoms of neurovascular compression (such as thoracic outlet syndrome). Working scalenes is indicated when there is numbness or tingling in the ulnar nerve distribution area (the small and ring fingers and medial hand, Figure 13.7), especially when symptoms worsen with forced inhalation (which engages the scalenes) or neck rotation (which scissors the brachial plexus between the anterior and medial scalenes, Figure 13.6).

Anterior Scalene Technique

These are all good reasons to include scalenes whenever you address the neck. However, working them directly can be tricky. The scalenes are often more contracted and denser than the tissues around them. Janda classifies the scalenes as "tonic" muscles, meaning that when stressed, they are prone to tightness rather than weakness, which may help explain why they're so often contracted (5). The scalenes also lie close to the sensitive nerves of the brachial plexus (Figure 13.5). This combination of hardness and proximity to nerves makes it difficult to use any degree of pressure or sliding, without causing referred nerve pain.

However, if we avoid sliding directly on the scalenes, and instead first slacken them by approximating their attachments, we can address the scalenes more comfortably and at much deeper levels. To accomplish this, begin by cradling your client's head in one hand (Figure 13.8). With the other hand, use the broad touch of several finger pads together to feel for the hard, longitudinally angled bellies of the anterior and medial scalenes, just above the clavicle and deep to the sternocleidomastoid. The hardest structure you feel here that isn't bone, is usually the anterior scalene.

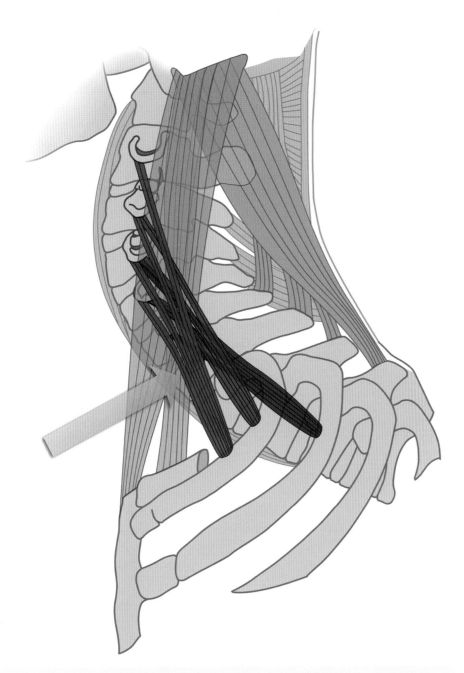

Figure 13.4
Although the anterior scalenes (arrow) are usually cervical flexors, when the neck is extended or lordotic their attachments move posterior to the vertebral bodies causing them to act as neck extensors, further perpetuating the lordosis when shortened.

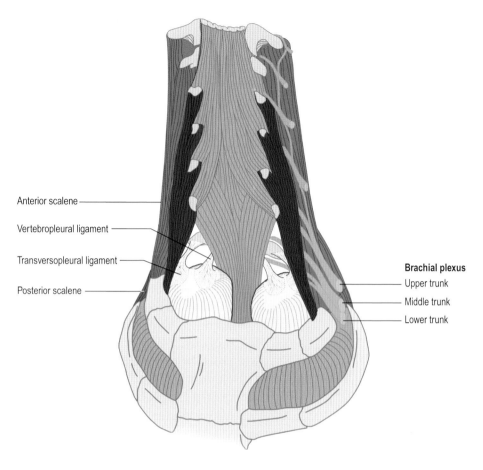

Anterior scalene

Vertebropleural ligament

Transversopleural ligament

Posterior scalene

Brachial plexus
Upper trunk
Middle trunk
Lower trunk

Figure 13.5
The nerves of the brachial plexus (yellow) pass between the anterior and medial scalenes.

Now lift the head, gently flexing the neck around the static fulcrum of your broad finger pads. You'll feel the bellies of the scalenes press against your fingers as you do this; apply just enough posterior pressure to resist the anterior movement of the scalenes and lower cervicals. This combination of vectors bends the anterior scalenes around your fulcrum hand, and encourages the cervicals to drop posteriorly, reducing their tendency towards anteriority (Figure 13.9).

If this feels "nervy" to your client, or especially if he or she feels tingling in the hands when you apply pressure, reposition your touch so that it is comfortable, usually by shifting slightly medially. Shift too far medially or too high, though, and you'll be near the carotid artery, jugular vein, or vagus nerve—none of which like direct pressure. Keep your touch broad, soft, and sensitive. It should never be uncomfortable to your client.

Once you have the counter-forces of neck flexion and posterior pressure comfortably in place, resist the temptation to slide, nudge, or otherwise move your fingers on the delicate scalenes. Instead, wait for the body to respond. After three to six breaths, you'll typically feel the scalenes and lower cervicals ease and drop posteriorly as the tissues soften and the nervous system adapts. This is the sign that it's okay to move to a new position.

By releasing and moving your fulcrum position (rather than by sliding), you can then work higher or lower parts of the scalenes. Feel for left/right asymmetries in the scalenes, and in the deeper plural ligaments (Figure 13.5) once the scalenes' tone is reduced. Alternatively, you can shift your fulcrum slightly laterally, adding

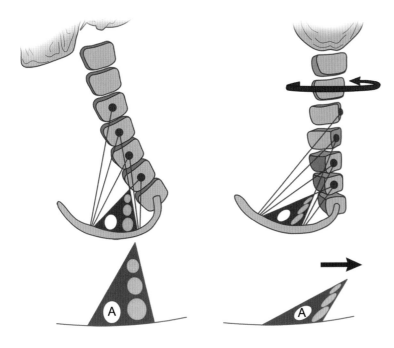

Figure 13.6
Neck rotation can "scissor" the brachial plexus and artery in the narrowing space between the scalenes.

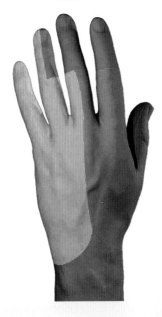

Figure 13.7
Compression of the brachial plexus by the scalenes or other structures can result in tingling, numbness, or weakness in the ulnar nerve distribution area (yellow).

a bit of cervical sidebending around your finger pads to access the medial and posterior scalenes (Figure 13.10). Wait for release and softening in each place. Stay in verbal contact with your client about any referred nerve pain. Be patient; wait for the release.

Of course, you'll want to work the scalenes only after you've done other preparatory work to warm up the outer layers of the neck (Chapter 11), and to accustom your client to your touch. Before you finish, be sure to work the scalenes on both sides; however, if you find asymmetrical patterns the amount of time you spend on each side will be different. Finish your scalene work with integrative, balancing, soothing techniques; even if you avoided pressing directly on the nerves of the brachial plexus, working the tonic scalenes can be sympathetically activating rather than parasympathetically calming.

Because the "Mother Cat" technique is calming and settling, and because it works both sides of the body rather than one side at a time, it is an ideal complement to scalene work.

Key points: Anterior Scalene Technique

Indications include:
- Neck mobility or positional asymmetries, including torticollis.
- Head-forward and "dowager's hump" postures.
- "Cold" whiplash injuries (Chapter 10).
- Respiratory issues, such as asthma or emphysema.
- Neurovascular compression symptoms, as in thoracic outlet syndrome.

Purpose
- Increase posterior mobility of lower cervical vertebrae and base of the neck.
- Differentiate and reduce the resting tonus of the scalenes.
- Decompress the neurovascular pathways between anterior and medial scalenes.

See video of the Anterior Scalene Technique at www.a-t.tv/wb04

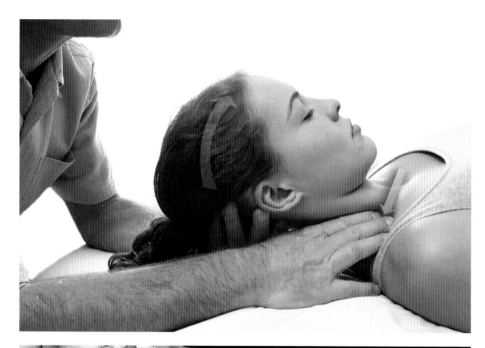

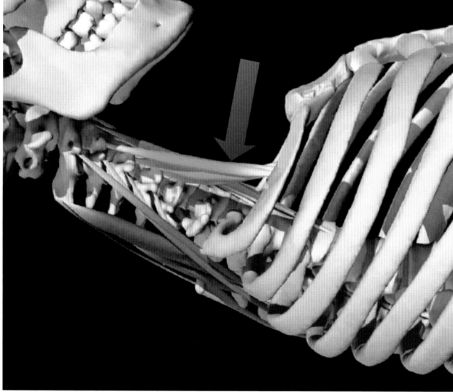

Figures 13.8/13.9

In the Anterior Scalene Technique, use a broad, soft touch to encourage the scalenes and lower cervical vertebrae to drop posteriorly (Figure 13.9), as you flex the neck in order to slacken the scalenes.

Instructions

After preparing outer layers of the neck:

1. Use a broad touch to gently press the anterior scalenes posteriorly, while using other hand to passively flex the neck around the fulcrum this touch provides.
2. Wait for 3–6 client breaths, feeling for tissues to soften, and for lower cervicals to drift posteriorly.
3. Returning neck to neutral position, moving fingers to a new position on the anterior scalenes, and repeat.
4. Variation: use gentle sidebending and shift your fingers laterally to work the medial and posterior scalenes.

Considerations

- Although very useful for cold whiplash, use caution with direct scalene work if hot whiplash signs are present to avoid worsening symptoms (Chapter 9).
- Avoid compressing nerves or vasculature. Communicate with client to ensure comfort.

"Mother Cat" Technique

You've seen what happens when a mother cat picks up her kitten by the scruff of its neck—the kitten goes limp (Figure 13.11). This reflex is the source of the name we've given this technique since humans also seem to let go, relax, and surrender with posterior traction on their neck fascia. Like a kitten being carried by its mother, people relax when their cervical fasciae are eased.

To perform the Mother Cat Technique, wrap a soft hand around the back of your supine client's neck, encompassing as much of both sides as possible (Figures 13.12–13.14). With the palm and fingers of your full hand, grasp and gather the outer layers of the nape of the neck straight backwards towards the posterior midline (that

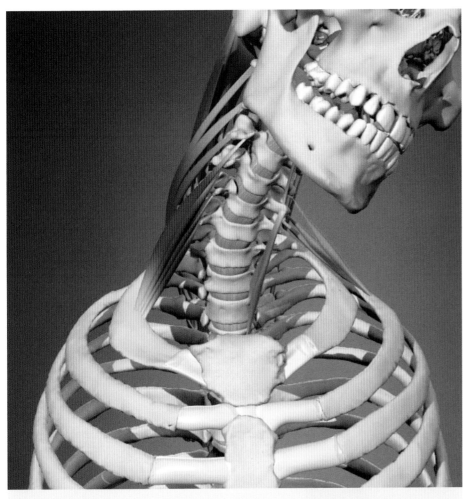

Figure 13.10

In a variation of the Anterior Scalene Technique, cervical sidebending allows access to the medial (red) and posterior (green) scalenes.

is, towards the floor), applying gentle posterior traction to the outer layers of the neck: the superficial and deep fasciae (Figure 13.15); and to the muscles within these outer layers, particularly trapezius. Allow the tissue layers to slowly slide out from under your hands a bit. Repeat several times, switching hands if you wish, although we're working both sides of the neck at the same time, the different shape of the left and right hands will allow you to access different aspects with each.

Our aim is to both ease and differentiate the outer tissues of the neck, and to shift the autonomic tone of our client's nervous system. Accordingly, let your pace be slow, steady, and patient as you repeat this technique, feeling for both tissue restrictions and for your client's parasympathetic relaxation response.

Although this technique's calming effects make it an ideal follow-up to the scalene work described earlier, these same properties make it an effective way to prepare a client for deep work as well. I originally learned this technique from William "Dub" Leigh, who called it "milking the neck," a name which hints at the repetitive, hypnotic motion that gives it its effectiveness. Dub, in turn, said he learned it from the legendary body therapy pioneer Moshe Feldenkrais, who (according to Dub) would patiently "milk the neck" for the first ten minutes of his hands-on Functional Integration sessions. Feldenkrais, a scrappy Ukrainian-Israeli physicist and Judo champion (who, incidentally, taught Israeli Prime Minister Ben-Gurion how to stand on his head), reportedly claimed that with just this technique and enough time, he "could have any man eating" out of his hand. If you're inclined to try this experiment, do let me know the results, but please remember, along with great power, comes great responsibility.

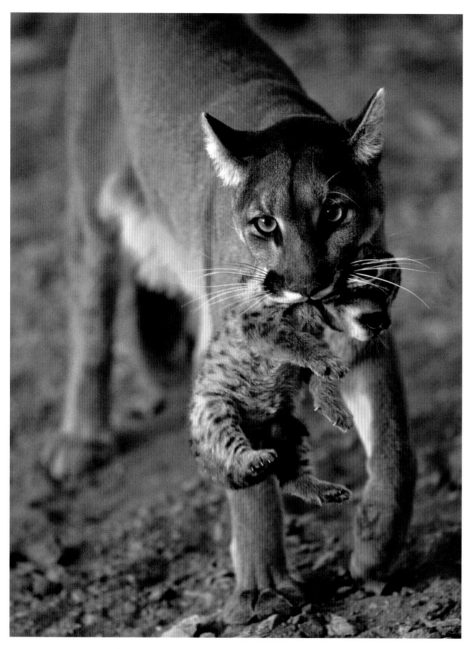

Figure 13.11

A female mountain lion carrying her kit by the skin, superficial, and deep fascia of the neck.

Key points: "Mother Cat" Technique

Indications include:

- Cervical mobility restrictions or pain.
- Autonomic sympathetic arousal.
- Useful before or after deeper, more focused neck work.

Purpose

- Prepare neck before deeper, more focused work.
- Increase elasticity and differentiation of outer layers of the neck.
- Regulate autonomic activation by increasing parasympathetic response.
- Integration and closure after deep cervical work.

Instructions

1. Gently gather outer layers of both sides of the posterior neck.
2. Apply slow, gentle traction posteriorly (towards the floor). Avoid producing any sensation of choking or unpleasant tightness across the front of the throat.
3. Allow the tissues to slowly glide from under your hand.
4. Reposition and repeat, entire posterior neck.

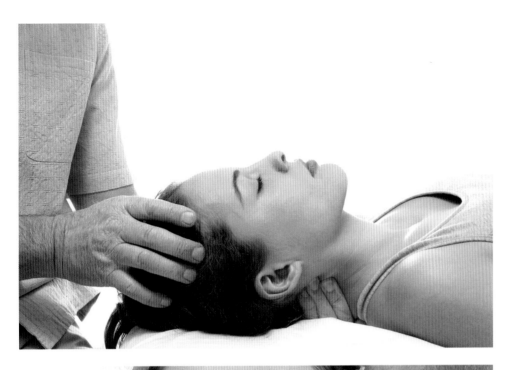

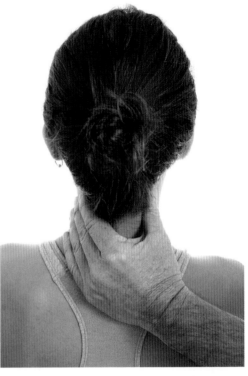

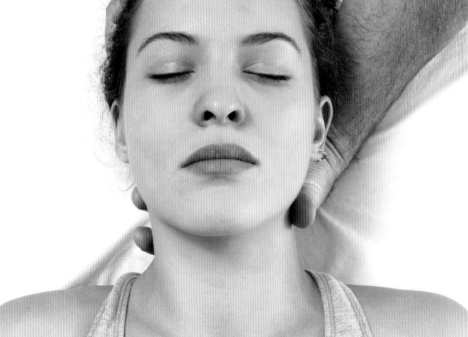

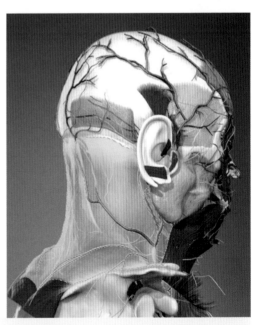

Figures 13.12/13.13/13.14/13.15

The "Mother Cat" Technique is an effective complement to scalene work, since it is bilateral, posterior, broad, superficial, and calming (in contrast to the scalene technique's one-sided, anterior, focused, deep, and stimulating characteristics). With your active hand, gently gather the superficial and deep cervical fascia (green, Figure 13.15) posteriorly; your other hand is simply monitoring and supporting.

References

[1] Anaritius, Anthony Lo Bello (2009) *The Commentary of Al-Nayrizi on Books II-IV of Euclid's Elements of Geometry*. Leiden: Brill. Xvi.

[2] Ivanichev, G.A. (1979) Anterior scalene muscle syndrome in spastic torticollis. *Klinicheskaia meditsina*. 57(9). p. 74–76.

[3] Goodman, C. and Snyder T. (2013) *Differential Diagnosis for Physical Therapists: Screening for Referral*. Elsevier Health Sciences.

[4] O'Rahilly, R. et al. (2008) *Basic Human Anatomy*. Dartmouth Medical School. 22(1).

[5] Janda, V. (1988) Muscles and cervicogenic pain syndromes. In: Ruth Grant, (ed). *Physical Therapy of the Cervical and Thoracic Spine*. New York: Churchill Livingstone.

[6] Leigh, W. (1984) Author's training notes.

Picture credits

Figures 13.1, 13.3, 13.7, 13.9, 13.10 and 13.15 courtesy Primal Pictures, used by permission.

Figure 13.2 Image courtesy Eric Franklin, originator of the Franklin Method (www.franklin-method.com), used by permission.

Figures 13.4, 13.5, 13.6, 13.8, 13.12, 13.13, and 13.14 courtesy AdvancedTrainings.com.

Figure 13.11 courtesy Thinkstock.

Study Guide

The Scalenes

1 **Working with the scalenes is indicated when there is numbness and tingling in which two fingers?**

a forefinger and middle finger (the "Peace Sign" sign)
b small and ring fingers
c thumb, forefinger, and middle finger
d forefinger and little finger (the "Horns Sign" sign)

2 **According to the text, in which of these cases would deep work on the scalenes be indicated?**

a as preparation or integration
b chronic, older injuries
c hot whiplash
d sympathetic ANS activation (fight or flight)

3 **What is the suggested direction of finger pressure in the Anterior Scalene Technique?**

a superior
b inferior
c posterior
d away from the practitioner

4 **Which word best describes the action of the practitioner's fulcrum hand in the Anterior Scalene Technique?**

a static
b gliding
c differentiating
d stripping

5 **According to the text, the LEFT scalenes would often be tighter in:**

a a left-handed person
b a right-handed person
c cold whiplash
d hot whiplash

For Answer Keys, visit www.Advanced-Trainings.com/v2key/

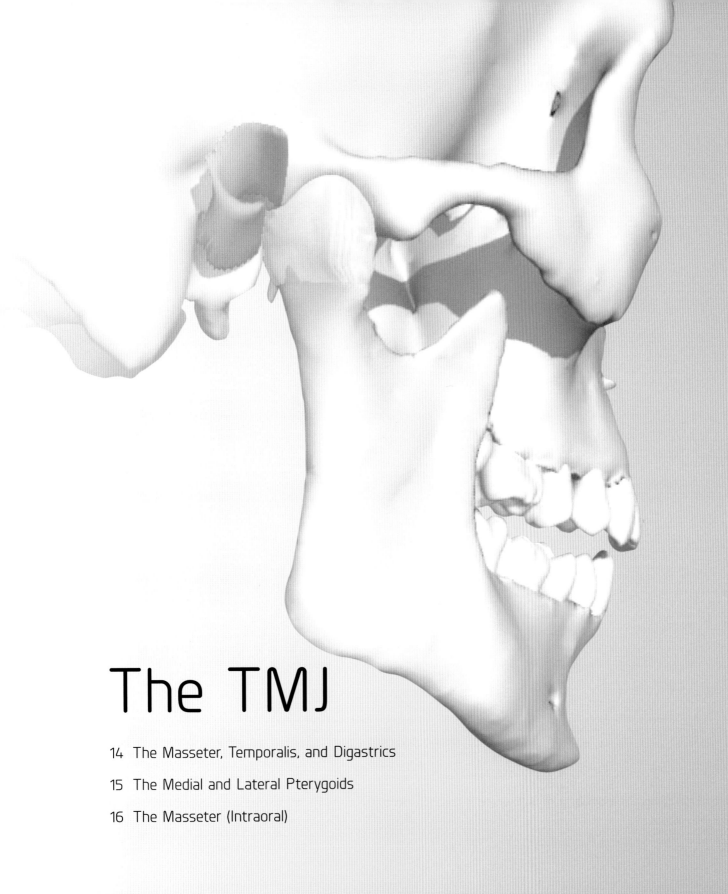

The TMJ

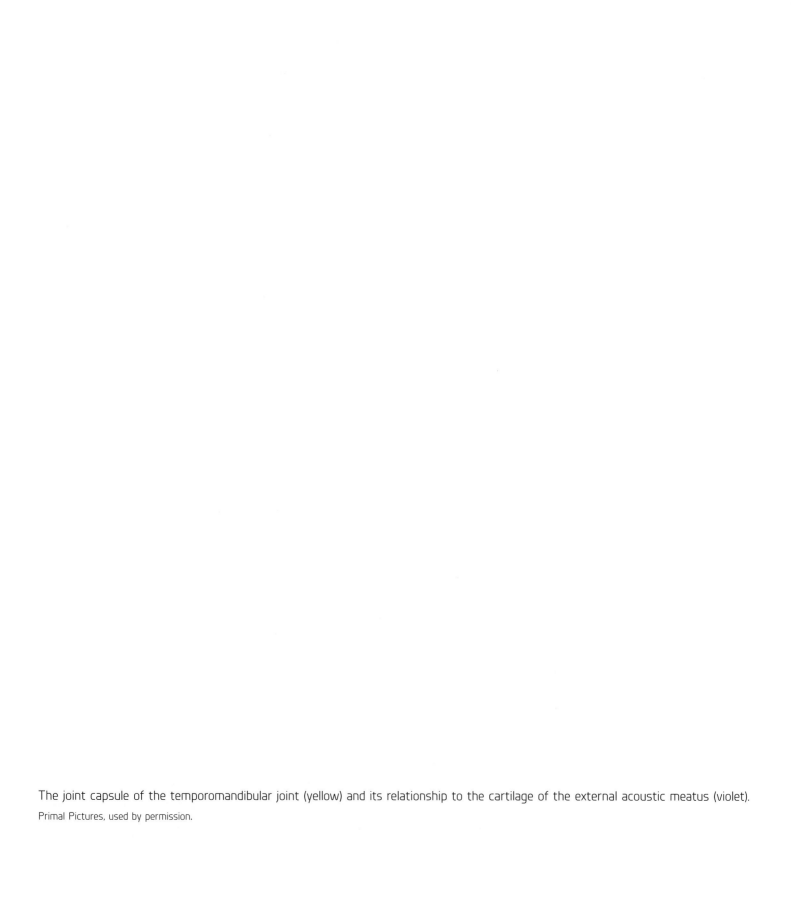

The joint capsule of the temporomandibular joint (yellow) and its relationship to the cartilage of the external acoustic meatus (violet).

Primal Pictures, used by permission.

The Masseter, Temporalis, and Digastrics

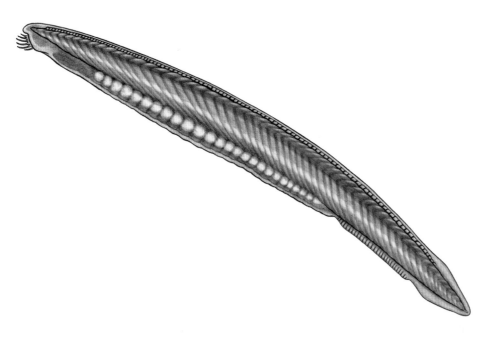

Figure 14.1

Amphioxus or lancelet, a small jawless fish-like invertebrate that is the closest living relative of the vertebrates.

Introduction: The Jaw and TMJ

Where would we be without our jaws? In the evolutionary version of our creation story, there was a long period when no animals had them. Ancient animals such as amphioxus had a mouth, but not a mandible (Figure 14.1). Once jaws appeared, however, they proved extremely popular, as all vertebrates (except for lampreys and hagfish) now have mandibles.

As useful as jaws are, they do come with complications. In modern humans, primary among these are Temporomandibular Joint and Muscle Disorders (TMJMD or TMD), or Temporomandibular Joint Syndrome. These umbrella terms describe conditions characterized by biting discomfort, jaw clicking, facial and jaw pain, earaches, headaches, gastric disturbance, and restricted jaw motion, among other symptoms. Although estimates of TMD prevalence range from about 5 percent (1 and 2) to 18 percent (3) of the populations studied, the percentage of people who experience TMD–like symptoms at some point in their lives is likely much higher. Women are most prone to TMD, with up to nine times more women than men seeking treatment (3).

This three-part section will look at several ways myofascial work can help jaw issues such as TMD. This initial chapter will present ways to assess and address important structures that influence the delicate balance of forces at the temporomandibular joints (TMJs)—specifically the masseters, temporalis, and digastrics. Chapter 15 will describe intraoral work with the pterygoids, often crucial to alleviating TMJ symptoms. Chapter 16 will discuss further ways to work with the masseters, and ways to close and integrate the jaw work in this section. As with the rest of the book, these techniques

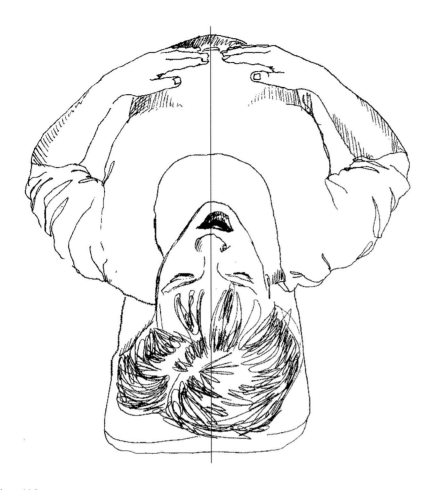

Figure 14.2
Assessing side-to-side jaw alignment. Look for lateral deviation anywhere in the cycle of depression/elevation.

can be incorporated into your work one by one, or this entire section can serve as a framework for a comprehensive jaw protocol.

Alignment, coordination, and myofascia

Think about it: the jaw hangs from the skull by soft tissue. While this allows the mobility we need to chew, speak, and swallow, it also makes the jaw vulnerable to misalignment. If the surrounding myofascial structures (outlined in Table 14.1, page 145) aren't differentiated or elastic enough to allow coordinated function, the movable jaw can easily be pulled out of line. The powerful forces of bite pressure compound the effects of this jaw misalignment, which can cause increased friction, compression, or binding of the articular discs and surrounding tissues (Figures 14.3 and 14.4). The result can be tissue irritation, pain, and if uncorrected, possible joint damage and degeneration over time.

Although the compression associated with jaw misalignment (Figures 14.5 and 14.6) is just one of the many issues that can contribute to temporomandibular joint pain and discomfort (4), it is a factor that we can readily address with our hands-on approach, and one that, in our experience, can make a significant difference in those suffering from TMD.

TMJ Tracking Technique

Assessment

From directly above your client's head, watch for side-to-side deviation of the jaw with gentle opening and closing (Figure 14.2). Don't ask your client to open the jaw past his or her point of comfort. If he or she has jaw pain, joint noises, or a history of temporomandibular joint dysfunction (TMJD), keep the opening and repetitions to a minimum. Toothpicks wedged in the gaps between the mesial (central) pair of teeth in both the upper and lower jaws can make any misalignment more obvious.

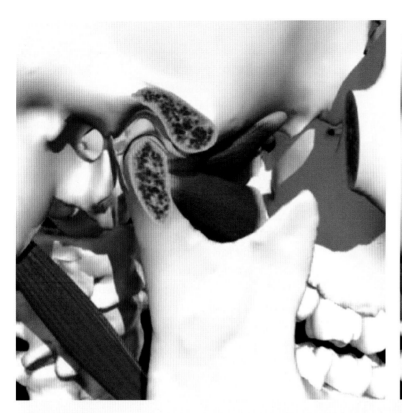
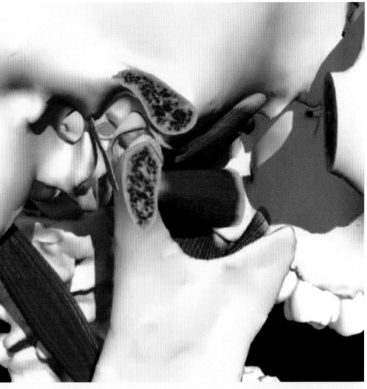

Figures 14.3/14.4

Phases of jaw opening (mandibular depression) at the temporomandibular joint (TMJ). Note how much the mandible drops forward and out of its condyle when opening. Notice also the mobility of the articular disc (in green). The disc floats within the joint capsule, and is positioned by articular membranes which are continuous with the lateral pterygoid anteriorly, and the membrane of the joint capsule posteriorly.

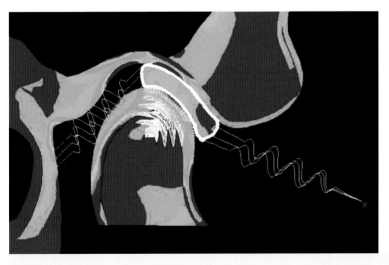
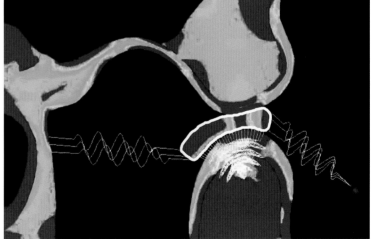

Figures 14.5/14.6

As the mandible slides forward in depression, the articular disc (outlined in white) is pulled into position by the articular membranes (thin zig-zag lines). Red indicates areas of highest compression (which can be exacerbated by misalignment or tension) in these computer-generated images.

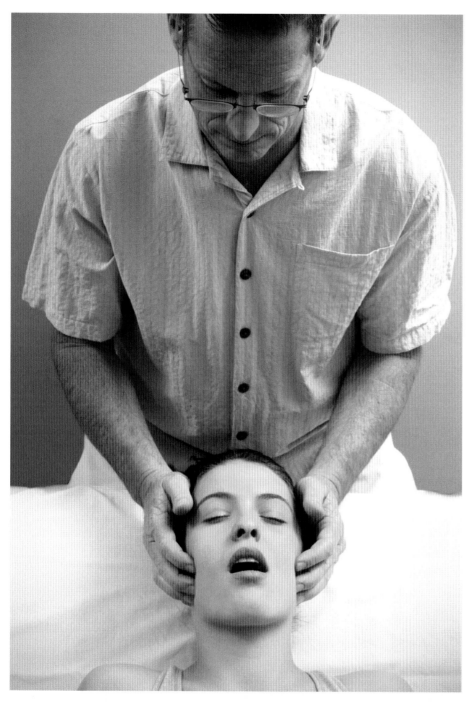

Figure 14.7

In the masseter portion of the TMJ Tracking Technique, feel for and release any asymmetrical contraction or shortening in the myofascia and muscular fibers of the masseters as your client opens (depresses) the jaw.

Masseter

As your client opens and closes the jaw, use your fingertips or palms to monitor the masseters and their surrounding fascia, comparing tissue movement of the left and right sides. Feel for any tissues that don't eccentrically lengthen or move caudally (inferiorly) during jaw opening. Feel particularly for any asymmetrical contraction or shortening in the myofascia and muscular fibers of the masseters (Figures 14.7 and 14.8) as the jaw moves. Stay away from glands or uncomfortable areas.

Coax any one-sided areas of tissue bunching or persistent contraction to release in a caudal (inferior) direction during opening; in other words, use your touch to encourage side-to-side balance of eccentric lengthening during jaw depression. Imagine letting out the reins on a horse that pulls to one side (Figure 14.9): it is the lengthening of the shorter rein that allows the horse's head back to the center, and to track straight.

As shown in Table 14.1, if the masseter is involved in jaw deviation, you'll generally feel tighter or less mobile tissues on the same side as the deviation (for example, the right masseter in Figure 14.2), but work whatever tissue or movement restrictions your hands find. Assess and work the entire masseter, staying alert for changes in the jaw's side-to-side tracking.

Temporalis

If you still see jaw deviation after working the masseter, the next step would be to use your fingertips to assess and work the temporalis and its broad fascia on the sides of the cranium (Figure 14.17 on p150) in the same way as you did the masseter. Use the client's active opening (depression) to encourage any thickened or undifferentiated temporalis tissues to lengthen in an eccentric, caudal direction. Keep monitoring

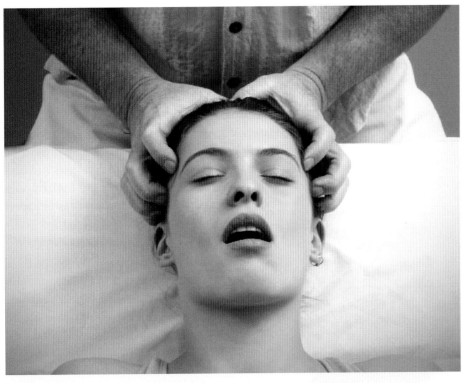

Figure 14.8
For the temporalis portion of the TMJ Tracking Technique, as your client opens and closes the jaw, use your fingertips to feel into the temporalis and its fascia. Feel for the various parts of the temporalis' contraction at different phases of opening and closing. Use your gentle pressure to release and balance any asymmetrical contractions.

Table 14.1 Myofascial Contributors to Jaw Deviation.

For lateral jaw deviation with elevation and depression, assess and work:

- Same-side masseter, temporalis, superficial fascia, and/or digastrics
- Opposite-side medial pterygoid; lateral pterygoid (particularly if deviation is upon initiation of depression). See Chapter 15.

For lateral jaw deviation with protrusion or retraction, assess and work:

- Any/all of above, particularly:
  Same-side digastric and posterior temporalis (since horizontal fibers there help retract the jaw, Figure 14.17).

the jaw for its tracking and feel for the various parts of the temporalis contracting at different phases of opening and closing (Figure 14.8).

In addition to lateral deviation, working the masseters and temporalis as described above can also be useful for working with other complaints, such as whiplash (Chapters 9 and 10); jaw tension and bruxism (Chapter 15); or tension headaches (Chapter 17) and migraines (Chapter 18).

The next step in our jaw-pain sequence is to apply the principles we used with elevation and depression to jaw protrusion and retraction.

Key points: TMJ Tracking Technique (Masseter and Temporalis)

Indications include:
- Lateral jaw deviation with depression and elevation.
- TMJD, TMJ pain, jaw tension, bruxism.
- Whiplash.
- Tension-type and migraine headaches.

Purpose
- Assess and release asymmetrical eccentric lengthening in masseter and/or temporalis.
- Coordinate and align depression and elevation jaw movements.

Instructions
1. Sitting above the client's head, watch for side-to-side deviations with gentle jaw opening and closing. (Hint: use toothpicks between the upper and lower teeth to reveal subtle misalignment).
2. Feel for any asymmetrical eccentric lengthening in the myofascia and muscular fibers of the masseters and temporalis.
3. Coax any areas that lack eccentric lengthen to move caudally (inferior) during jaw opening.

Movements
- Active jaw depression and elevation.

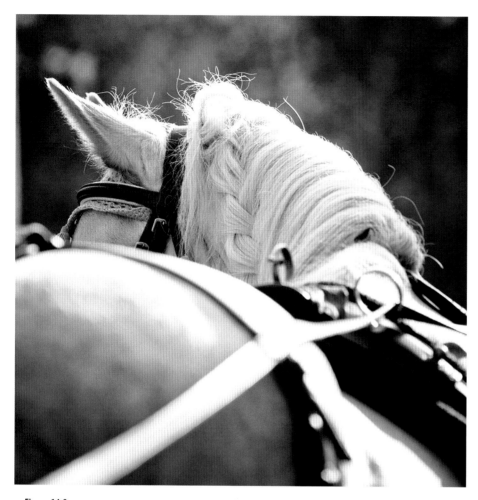

Figure 14.9

Like letting out the reins on a horse that pulls to one side, the direction of your pressure will be downward or inferior in the TMJ Tracking Technique, since it is the lengthening of the shorter rein that allows the horse's head back to the center, and to track straight.

The Digastrics

Next, we'll focus on the digastric ("two-bellied") muscles, which play an equally important role in jaw pain, alignment, and balanced motion. Because the digastrics both depress (open) and retract the jaw, if one digastric is tighter, less differentiated, or less elastic than the other, it will pull the jaw homolaterally (towards its same side) when the jaw moves. Bilaterally tight digastrics can also force the mandible posteriorly in the TMJ, causing jamming and compression at the posterior aspect of that joint—a frequent site of TMJ pain.

First, a quick anatomy review: the digastrics' left and right anterior bellies form much of the floor of the mouth. They have a sling-like connection to the hyoid bone via central tendons, continue posteriorly with a second belly, and then attach to the medial aspect of the mastoid processes, just behind the ear (Figure 14.11).

Anterior Digastric Technique

Begin by reassessing your client's jaw alignment, this time while your client actively protrudes and retracts the jaw. While looking from above as in the previous assessment, ask your client to "Gently slide your jaw forwards," like a bulldog. You should see the jaw slide straight forwards, vs. being pulled to the left or right. If you see signs of lateral deviation, the digastric on the same side is a likely factor.

By wrapping your fingertips around the inferior border of the jaw (Figure 14.12), gently lengthen the anterior bellies of the digastrics and the floor of mouth by working in a posterior direction. Use your client's slow, active protrusion and side-to-side movements to slide the digastrics past your fingers, rather than a gliding touch. This will allow your client to control the pace and intensity of the sensation, as well providing some neuromuscular re-education from the active movement. Feel for any tissue restriction

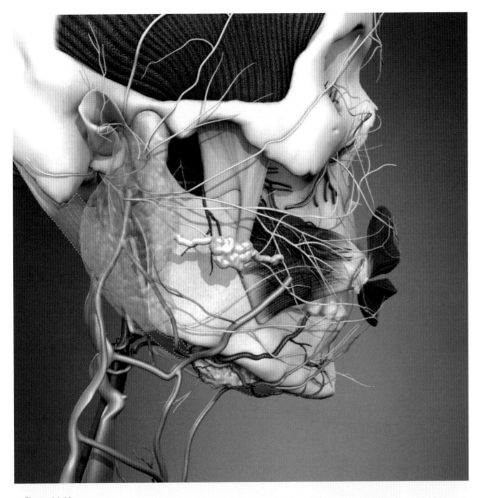

Figure 14.10

Glands, nerves, lymph nodes, vessels, and other delicate structures surround the posterior digastric bellies, so we work them via their more available posterior attachment on the mastoid process.

on the same side of any jaw deviation. Optionally, add active opening (mandibular depression). Continue working posteriorly as far as the hyoid bone (where the structures of the anterior neck meet the floor of the mouth). Be detailed and thorough, but use caution around the glands in this area: stay on fascia, muscle, and bone.

Key points: Anterior Digastric Technique

Indications include:
- Posterior TMJ pain.
- Same-side deviation of jaw with opening.
- Lateral jaw movement with protrusion and retraction.

Purpose
- Aligned jaw motion in protrusion and retraction.

Instructions
1. Fingers wrap around the inferior border of the jaw into the anterior bellies of the digastrics.
2. Cue the client's slow, active movement.

Movements
- Slow, active protrusion or depression to slide the digastrics past the practitioner's static, sensitive touch.

Precaution
- Avoid delicate glands in this area—stay on muscle, bone, and fascia.

Posterior Digastric Technique

Since glands, nerves, and other delicate structures surround the posterior digastrics (see Figure 14.10), we won't try to work their posterior bellies with direct pressure. Instead, we'll shift their resting tone via a Golgi reflex response. With a firm but sensitive touch, press into the attachments of the posterior digastrics on the anteromedial aspect of the mastoid process (Figure 14.13). Cue your client to slide the jaw forward (protrusion, Figure 14.14); this will allow you to more precisely locate the digastrics'

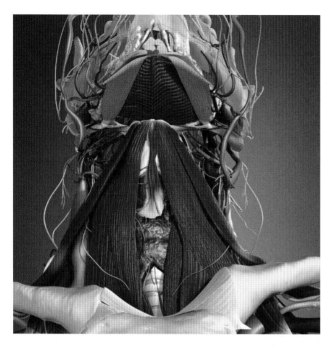

Figure 14.11

The digastrics' left and right anterior bellies (in green) form much of the floor of the mouth. After a sling-like connection to the hyoid bone via central tendons, they continue posteriorly with a second belly. The mandible is transparent in this view.

See video of the Posterior Digastric Technique at www.a-t.tv/ta07

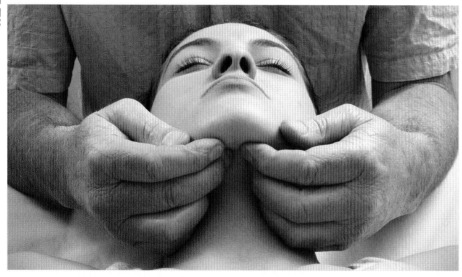

Figure 14.12

The Anterior Digastric Technique. Use your client's slow, active protrusion and side-to-side movements to gently slide the digastrics past your fingers. Feel for tissue inelasticity on the same side of any jaw deviation. Use caution around the glands in this area.

attachments. To familiarize yourself with the precise angle and pressure needed, try this technique on yourself before attempting it on a client.

Once you locate both posterior digastric attachments on the mastoid processes, have your client repeat the active protrusion, alternating it with active jaw retraction (Figure 14.15). It can be helpful to combine retraction with work on the posterior temporalis as well, since this section of the fan-shaped temporalis is also involved in jaw retraction. Jaw depression (opening, Figure 14.16) is also useful as an alternate way to activate the digastrics.

When stimulated with a combination of pressure and active movement, the Golgi tendon organs (which are concentrated around muscles' tendinous attachments) signal the digastrics' alpha motor neurons to lower the muscles' firing rate. This results in a reduction in tone in the entire muscle (Figure 14.16), and finer movement coordination overall (5).

Key points: Posterior Digastric Technique

Indications include:
- Posterior TMJ pain.
- Same-side deviation of jaw with opening.
- Lateral jaw movement with protrusion and retraction.

Purpose
- Align jaw motion in protrusion and retraction.

Instructions
1. Locate posterior digastric attachments on the anteromedial aspect of the mastoid processes by cueing active jaw protrusion and retraction.
2. Working bilaterally, use gentle pressure on posterior digastrics' attachments in combination with active protrusion, retraction, and depression.
3. Repeat, feeling for the subtle softening and tonus shift that indicates a Golgi tendon organ response.

Movements
- Slow, focused active jaw protrusion, retraction, and depression.

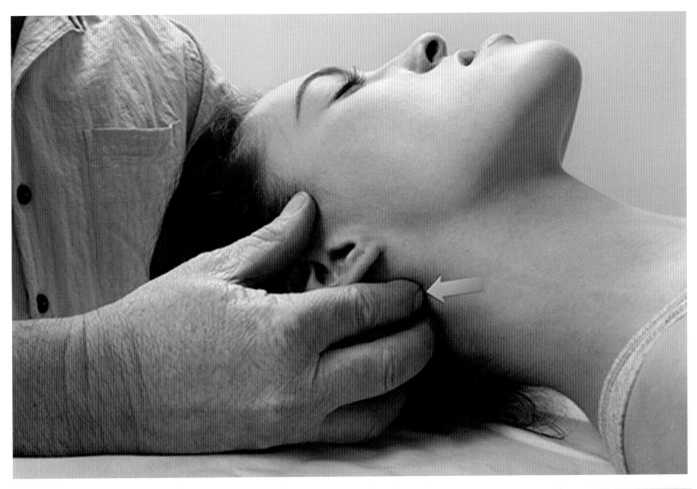

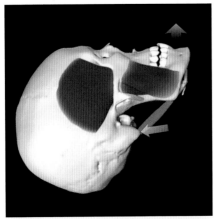
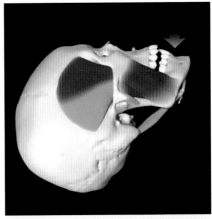
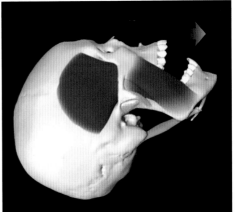

Figures 14.13/14.14/14.15/14.16

The Posterior Digastric Technique. Gentle but firm static pressure on the digastrics' posterior attachments (on the medial aspect of the mastoid processes; violet arrow) in combination with active jaw protrusion (Figure 14.16), retraction (Figure 14.17), and depression (Figure 14.18) changes the digastrics' resting tone via a Golgi tendon organ response.

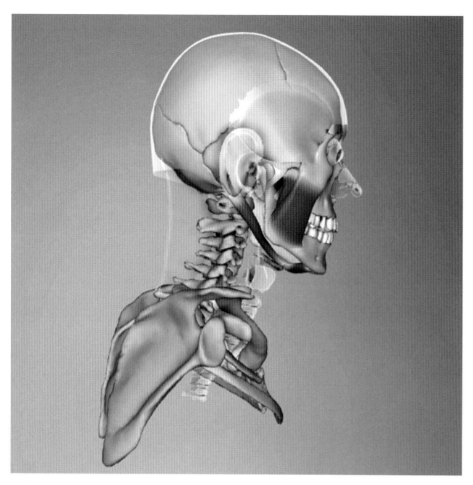

Figure 14.17

Since the temporalis and masseter are some of the larger, stronger, and more superficial structures crossing the TMJ, we address these first when working with jaw misalignment. The temporalis muscle is covered by the tough temporalis fascia (blue). The digastric muscles and hyoid bone are also pictured.

Indications

Assess and balance the digastrics whenever addressing TMJ and jaw issues, especially when you see jaw retraction, misalignment, or your client reports pain around the posterior TMJ. Of course, there can be additional causes of chronic mandibular retraction and posterior TMJ pain, such as a head-forward posture, tongue and throat constriction, superficial fascial restrictions, and postural influences from the rest of the body; however, you'll find that working with the digastrics is an essential technique to have in your TMJ toolbox.

TMJ pain can have many contributing factors. TMD is often multi-factorial, with mind-body, stress, pain perception, and other complex factors all contributing. Physically, head-forward postures (6), dental issues, and back and pelvic patterns (7) have all been correlated to TMJ pain.

However, even with all of these complexities, your clients will often report positive changes from just this simple tracking technique. If you see improvement, explore your client's proprioceptive, inside-out experience of sensation with jaw movement. The proprioceptive learning involved will help to give your client more options if pain or tension returns.

On the other hand, if you still see side-to-side deviation after the masseter and temporalis tracking, or if your client has persistent TMJ pain, don't be discouraged. Your next step will be work with other, deeper structures crossing the TMJ (Table 14.1). The following chapters offer some techniques for doing this.

References

[1] Isong, U., Gansky, S.A., and Plesh, O. (2008) Temporomandibular joint and muscle disorder-type pain in U.S. adults: The National Health Interview Survey. *Journal of Orofacial Pain*. Fall, 22(4). p. 317–322.

[2] Deng, Y.M., Fu, M.K., and Hägg, U. (1995) Prevalence of temporomandibular joint dysfunction (TMJD) in Chinese children and adolescents: A cross-sectional epidemiological study. *European Journal of Orthodontics*.17(4). p. 305–309. Review. PubMed PMID: 8521924.

[3] Levitt, S.R. and McKinney, M.W. (1994) Validating the TMJ scale in a national sample of 10,000 patients: Demographic and epidemiologic characteristics. *Journal of Orofacial Pain*. 8 p. 25–35.

[4] Scrivani, S.J., Keith, D.A., and Kaban, L.B. (2008) Temporomandibular disorders. *The New England Journal of Medicine*. p. 2693–2705.

[5] Schleip, R. (2003) Fascial plasticity: A new neurobiological explanation, Part I. *Journal of Bodywork and Movement Therapies*. 7(1). p. 14.

[6] Andrade, A.V., Gomes, P.F., and Teixeira-Salmela, L.F. (2007) Cervical spine alignment and hyoid bone positioning with temporomandibular disorders. *Journal of Oral Rehabilitation*. 34. p. 767–772.

[7] Cuccia, A. and Caradonna, C. (2009) The relationship between the stomatognathic system and body posture. *Clinics (Sao Paulo)*. 64(1). p. 61–66. http://www.scielo.br/pdf/clin/v64n1/a11v64n1.pdf. [Accessed December 2015]

Picture credits

Figure 14.1 Artist: Giovanni Maki. Used under the terms of the Creative Commons Attribution License.

Figure 14.2 is from the copyrighted "Range-of-Motion Testing" charts by R. Finn and C.M. Shiffett, used by permission.

Figures 14.3, 14.4, 14.10, 14.11, and 14.14–18 courtesy Primal Pictures, used by permission.

Figures 14.5 and 14.6 courtesy Dr. J.W. DeVocht, used by permission.

Figures 14.7, 14.8, 14.12, and 14.13 courtesy Advanced-Trainings.com.

Figure 14.9 Thinkstock.

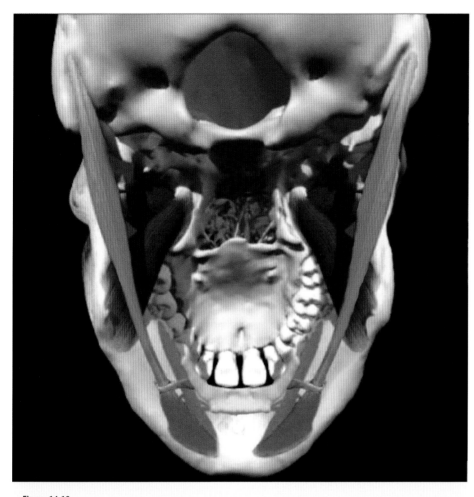

Figure 14.18

The digastrics from below. Their bilateral arrangement means they play an important role in jaw alignment and balanced motion. Use the Anterior and Posterior Digastric Techniques when you see lateral deviation with protrusion or depression.

Study Guide

The Masseter, Temporalis, and Digastrics

1 **What are the actions of the digastrics?**

a laterally move and retract the jaw
b depress the jaw and protract the jaw
c elevate and protract the jaw
d depress and retract the jaw

2 **What is the stated rationale for working the masseter and temporalis first?**

a no rationale was given for working the masseter and temporalis first
b the most trigger points are typically found in these muscles
c they are more important in jaw alignment than other muscles
d they are larger and more superficial than other jaw muscles

3 **What is a Golgi tendon response?**

a it is a parasympathetic response when stimulating a tendon
b it is a spinal reflex that facilitates the motor neuron's synapse
c It is a spinal reflex that lowers the muscles' firing rate
d it is a protective tightening of a tendon's muscle fibers

4 **According to the text, why is the Golgi tendon organ response used to work the posterior digastrics?**

a to add variety to techniques used
b to avoid pressure on glands, lymph nodes, and nerves
c the anterior digastric does not readily respond to the Golgi reflex, but the posterior digastric does
d no reason was given

5 **What can happen when the right-side digastric is tighter than the left?**

a the jaw can close first on the left
b the jaw can be pulled to the left
c the jaw can close first on the right
d the jaw can be pulled to the right

For Answer Keys, visit www.Advanced-Trainings.com/v2key/

The Pterygoids

An important first step when addressing jaw pain or temporomandibular joint dysfunction (TMD) is to improve differentiation and coordination of the larger, more superficial structures affecting the jaw, as described in the previous chapter. If jaw pain or misaligned movement persists after thoroughly performing those techniques, the next step would be to address the intraoral structures (those inside the mouth) that might be contributing to the misalignment. In this chapter, I'll describe ways to work with the medial and lateral pterygoids, both important players in jaw health, although each for different reasons, as we shall see.

Both the medial and lateral pterygoids are deep structures, and although there are ways to access portions of them from outside the mouth, in our experience, working intraorally (with client permission) is the most effective way to address both. Before working inside the mouth, be sure to explain the purpose and intention of the work, and obtain explicit permission from your client to work within his or her mouth.[1] Most clients are very receptive to intraoral work when they understand what it entails, and why it is being proposed.

Medial pterygoids

The medial pterygoids are powerful muscles, and since TMJ health is dependent on coordinated function of its supporting soft tissues, working these structures is indicated whenever you see symptoms of TMD.

It is useful to think of the medial pterygoids as the "inside masseters" of the mouth. Like the masseters, medial pterygoids are strong elevators (closers) of the jaw. Together, the medial pterygoids and masseters create a pair of V-shaped slings (Figure 15.1) on either side of the mouth

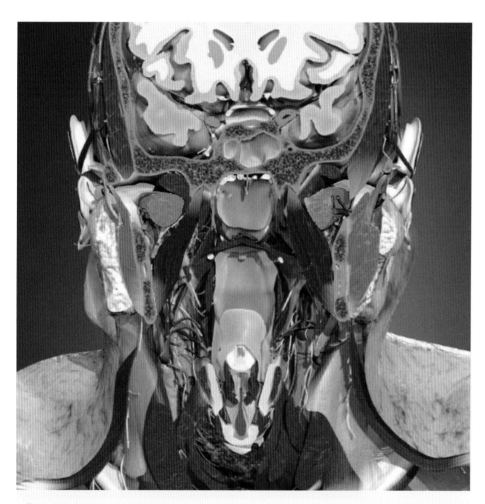

Figure 15.1

Coronal cross-section, showing the pterygoids. The medial pterygoids (purple) together with the masseters (orange) form two V-shaped "slings" that support, close, and help align the mandible. Also shown are the lower head of the lateral pterygoids (green) and the articular surfaces of the TMJ (yellow).

1 Some states or governing agencies put stipulations or limitations on manual therapy practitioners' work within the mouth, such as requiring specific training or endorsements, and a few prohibit intraoral work outright. In addition to getting your clients' explicit consent, be sure to be familiar with your local scope-of-practice regulations and requirements.

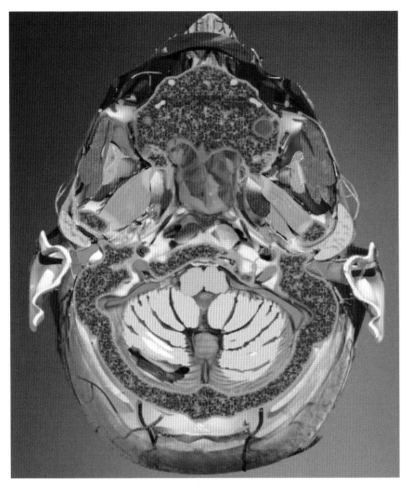

Figure 15.2

Horizontal cross-section, showing the lower head of the lateral pterygoids (green), the upper attachments of hte medial pterygoids (purple), the masseters (orange), temporalis (pink), and the articular surfaces of the TMJ (yellow).

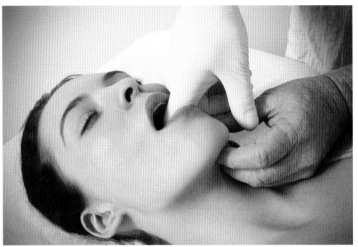

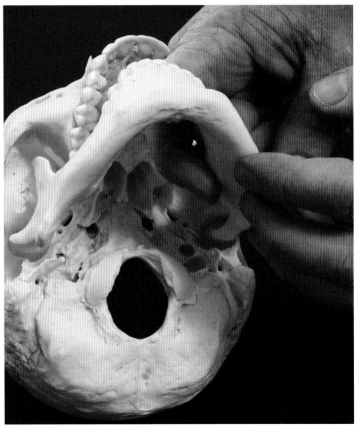

Figures 15.3/15.4

To work the medial pterygoids, gently press into their lower attachments on the medial aspect of the jaw, from both inside and outside the mouth simultaneously. Using sensitive, static pressure, ask your client to make small, slow jaw movements to help you locate the attachments, and to facilitate release.

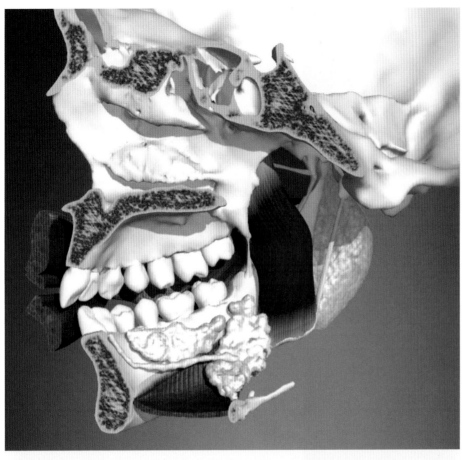

Figure 15.5

When working the medial pterygoid (purple), keep in mind that it is surrounded by nerves, salivary and parotid glands, and the delicate mucous membranes under the tongue.

that support, align, and elevate the jaw. Habitual tension or left/right imbalance here can exert inappropriate force on the TMJ, contributing to irritation and dysfunction. The medial pterygoid's uppermost attachments on the sphenoid bone are high and deep in the soft palate, and are probably impossible to palpate directly (Figure 15.2). However, the belly and inferior attachments of the muscles are easily accessible where they line the inside of the jaw, like a mirror-image of the masseter's outside position (Figure 15.1).

Medial Pterygoid Technique

To work the medial pterygoid, gently palpate its belly on the medial (inside) aspect of the jaw, while simultaneously feeling its inferior attachment outside the mouth, just inside the jaw's lower margin (Figures 15.3 and 15.4). Feel for areas of fascial inelasticity or higher myofascial density within the muscle belly, and especially at the lower attachments. Use care not to mistake the glands and other delicate structures here (Figure 15.5) for areas of myofascial density or tension. Some clients can have a mild gag reflex in this area, so work slowly and cautiously. Ask your client to make small, slow jaw movements (including protrusion, since that is one of the medial pterygoids' functions) to help you distinguish the inferior attachments just inside the mandible's angle, as it is at the attachments where the Golgi tendon organs are most concentrated. As mentioned elsewhere, steady pressure on Golgi tendon organs, combined with active movement, can influence the postural reflexes that govern the resting tone of the entire muscle group. Our intentions are lowered muscle tone, bilateral coordination, and greater myofascial adaptability, so encourage your client to relax the jaw, face, and neck, and to breathe, while you keep your pressure steady, slow, and receptive.

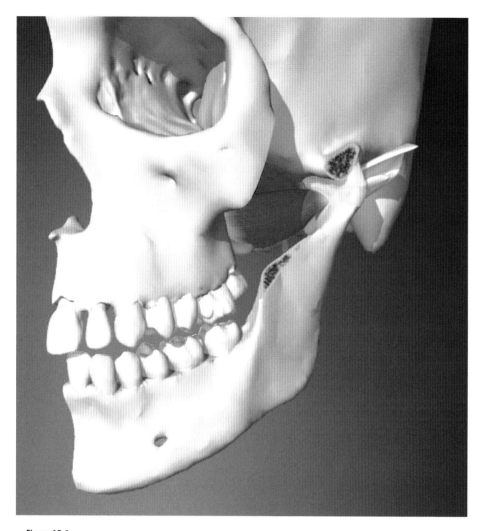

Figure 15.6

The lateral pterygoid (green) is in a unique position to both pull the jaw forward, and to influence the position of the TMJ's articular disc, as its superior head attaches to the TMJ capsule (yellow) and to the articular disc within. The zygomatic arch and the coronoid process of the mandible have been removed in this view to better show the lateral pterygoid.

Work both left and right medial pterygoids, spending more time on the denser or less elastic side.

Incidentally, the brain dedicates even more of its somatosensory cortex to the mouth, than it does to our hands. This means that the mouth may be the only place we work where your client feels your touch more acutely than you feel their tissue. Be extremely sensitive and patient when working intraorally. It is crucially important to practice the intraoral techniques on yourself first to get a sense of the kind of touch needed, and to experience the feeling of openness and ease afterwards.

Key points: Medial Pterygoid Technique

Indications include:
- Lateral jaw deviation with depression, elevation, and/or protrusion.
- TMJD, TMJ pain, jaw tension, bruxism.
- Whiplash.
- Tension-type and migraine headaches.

Purpose
- Reduce any medial pterygoid contributions to TMJ compression and misalignment by shifting medial pterygoid resting tone, coordinating their bilateral function, and increasing their myofascial adaptability.

Instructions
1. Use gentle pressure on one side's medial pterygoid simultaneously from inside and outside the mouth. Ask for active movement to locate muscle belly with inside hand, and inferior attachments with outside hand.
2. Hold these places as client continues slow, active movement. Feel for subtle shift in myofascial tonus.

Movements
- Slow, active jaw depression, elevation, protrusion, and retraction.

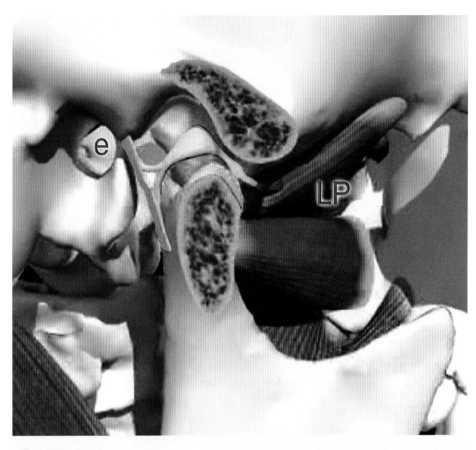

Figure 15.7

As the jaw opens (depresses), membranes contiguous with the TMJ capsule and the upper head of the lateral pterygoid ("LP") help position the articular disc within the joint (yellow). When there is jaw tension, misalignment, or excessive compression, the disc can be displaced (most often anteriorly, in the direction of lateral pterygoid pull). Note also that the anterior aspect of the external acoustic meatus ("e") forms the posterior side of the TMJ capsule.

Lateral pterygoids

The lateral pterygoid muscles affect TMJ health in at least three important ways. First, these paired muscles initiate jaw opening. Since their lower heads insert on the mandibular condyle (Figures 15.6 and 15.7), they pull the jaw anteriorly in order to begin the movement of jaw depression. If one side's lateral pterygoid is tighter (has a higher resting tone) than the other's, this can result in asymmetrical firing, and will misalign the jaw's movement upon initiation of opening.

The lateral pterygoid also affects the TMJ in a second way. As you open and close your mouth, the TMJ's articular disc is positioned by its suspensory membrane, which has fibers contiguous (directly attached) to the upper head of the lateral pterygoid (Figures 15.6 and 15.7). In a healthy joint, this helps keep the disc in position to cushion the contact point between the mandibular condyle and the temporal bone during opening and closing. However, tension in the lateral pterygoids can anteriorly displace the articular disc (4), the most common direction of displacement in TMD. When this happens, or when there is excessive compression on the disc, the condyle can slide on and off the disc during jaw movement, producing the pop or click often associated with TMD. In more severe cases, the disc remains anterior to the condyle; the telltale popping sound is absent, but jaw opening is painful and limited.

The third (but arguably the most significant way) that the lateral pterygoids affect TMJ health is their role as proprioceptors of jaw function. As you will experience when you try the technique below on yourself, the lateral pterygoids are extremely sensitive. This sensitivity reflects their rich concentration of mechanoreceptors that constantly monitor jaw position, movement, tension, and sensation (including pain). These small, deep, very sensitive muscles could be thought of as paired sensory organs, helping coordinate jaw movements and myofascial tension around the TMJs.

Lateral Pterygoid Technique

Assessment

Since the anterior wall of the ear canal is contiguous with the posterior side of the TMJ capsule (Figures 15.7 and 15.8), we can easily assess anterior mandibular condyle movement here. With your client's permission, position the tip of your little finger just inside each ear passage (Figures 15.9 and 15.10). With your finger pads, feel for the mandibular condyles, which are palpable on the anterior wall of the canal. Ask your client to slowly begin to open his or her jaw, and you'll feel the condyles glide anteriorly. As the jaw begins to open, which condyle glides anteriorly (away from your finger pad) first? The lateral pterygoid on that side is likely to have a higher resting tone, and so fires sooner or stronger than the other side. Begin by working that tighter side as described below, and then recheck.

Technique

Because the lateral pterygoids can be difficult to palpate (5), explore this area in your own mouth before attempting this work with a client. Using your little finger, slide along the outside of your upper teeth until you come to the back edge of the last molar. Laterally, feel the inside of your cheek for a vertical bony fin—this is the coranoid process of the mandible, and the strong temporalis tendon. You can confirm you're on the coranoid process by opening and closing your jaw slightly—the process will clearly move. Now shift your jaw to the same side (Figure 15.11) to open up more space between the coranoid process and the teeth. Notice that a small pocket opens up behind the last molar (Figure 15.12). You may have to open your mouth a bit more to feel this,

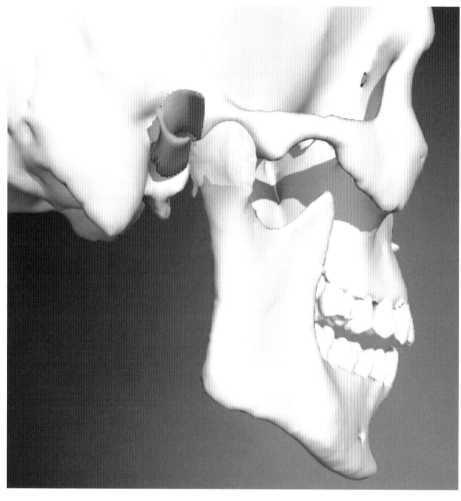

Figure 15.8

The anterior wall of the external acoustic meatus (purple) is contiguous with the posterior side of the TMJ capsule (yellow). Palpating the movement of the condyle just inside the ear canal is an effective way to assess lateral pterygoid tension and bilaterally balanced function.

but only do so enough to accommodate your finger as you move it further posteriorly and slightly medially. The tip of your finger will now be on the lateral pterygoid, which will often be softer or more sensitive than its surrounding structures. Confirm and refine your location by opening your jaw slightly and feeling the muscle contract.

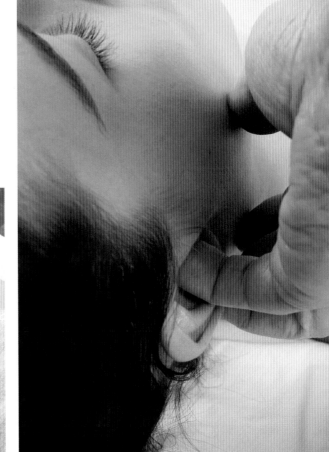

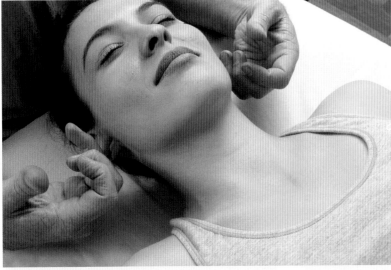

Figures 15.9/15.10

To assess left-right balance of the lateral pterygoids, use your finger pads to palpate the anterior wall of the external acoustic meatus. Feel for any left/right differences in the anterior movement of the mandibular condyles as the jaw begins to open. The tighter lateral pterygoid will typically be on the side that moves earlier or more.

Use the same approach with your clients, being very gentle, patient, and specific. Address the tighter side first, based on your assessment of condyle movement initiation, as described above. Apply steady, slow, receptive touch to the lateral pterygoid while asking for small opening and closing movements to facilitate a shift of its resting tone. Remember the lateral pterygoids' role as sense organs: they are very sensitive, and you don't need to stay here long.

Reassess condyle motion to see if the left and right mandibular condyles' anterior glide are now more coordinated, and check in with your client about any changes in pain level or their

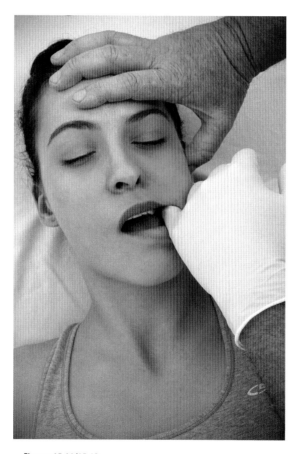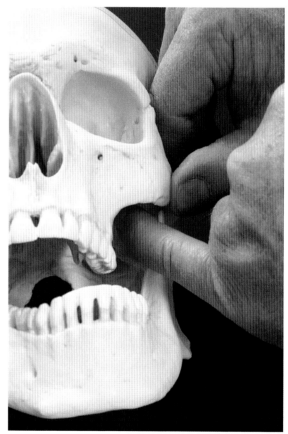

Figures 15.11/15.12

To access the sensitive lateral pterygoid, ask your client to shift their jaw towards the side you're working, and slide your finger posteriorly and slightly medially. Work here can reduce tension that can contribute to the anterior disc displacement characteristic of TMD, because the lateral pterygoid inserts on the TMJ capsule and the suspensory membrane of the articular disc.

own perception of movement. You may need to repeat on the same side, or work back and forth between the two lateral pterygoids to achieve more balanced movement and greater comfort.

Key points: Lateral Pterygoid Technique

Indications include:

- Lateral jaw deviation or uneven initiation of jaw depression, as assessed at the external acoustic meatuses.
- TMJD, TMJ pain, jaw tension, bruxism.

Purpose

- Coordinate and align the initiation of jaw opening by refining pterygoid proprioception and balancing any asymmetrical resting tone.
- Reduce any excessive lateral pterygoid tone, which might contribute anterior displacement of the TMJ's articular disc.

Instructions

1. After obtaining client permission, assess coordination of left/right mandibular condyle motion just inside external acoustic meatuses.
2. Begin with side that moved first (since it likely has earlier Lateral Pterygoid firing or higher resting tone).
3. Ask client to shift jaw to the same side to make room to facilitate access to the lateral pterygoid.
4. Using little finger, follow the outside of the upper teeth to the lateral pterygoid, just posterior to the the last molar.
5. Optionally, ask for small movements of active jaw depression.
6. Reassess condyle motion; repeat or work other side as needed in order to improve symmetry of jaw depression initiation.

Movements

- Same-side lateral deviation to allow access to lateral pterygoid.
- Slow, small jaw depression and elevation to facilitate placement, proprioception, and shift in resting tone.

Team players

Although the medial and lateral pterygoid techniques are often some of the "most valuable players" in your TMD lineup, they are by no means the entire team. Like star players, their key role can overshadow the importance of other structures and relationships. In dealing with most clients' temporomandibular joint (TMJ) symptoms, other structures and patterns will almost always need to be addressed as well. You can maximize your effectiveness by attending to other jaw-specific local factors, such as jaw alignment (Chapter 14), jaw tension (Chapter 16), bite occlusion, and cervical issues (Chapters 11–13). And it is also important to keep in mind the larger, global, whole-body patterns that affect the jaw too; issues such as pelvic tension (6), pelvic angle (7), and spinal curves (8) have all been shown to correlate with jaw function.

When you get the "most valuable players" of the pterygoids working together as a team with the rest of the body, the chances are very good that your clients with TMJ symptoms will feel much better, and you'll enjoy knowing that you've helped make that possible.

See video of the Lateral Pterygoid Technique at www.a-t.tv/tb05

References

[1] Schleip, R. (2003) Fascial plasticity: A new neurobiological explanation, Part I. *Journal of Bodywork and Movement Therapies.* 7(1). p. 11–19.

[2] Mehta, N.R. (2014) Internal temporomandibular joint derangement. *Merck Manuals Professional Edition.* http://www.merckmanuals.com/professional/dental-disorders/temporomandibular-disorders/internal-temporomandibular-joint-derangement. [Accessed December 2015]

[3] Christensen, L.V. and Troest, T. (1975) Clinical kinesthetic experiments on the lateral pterygoid muscle and temporomandibular joint in man. *Scandinavian Journal of Dental Research.* 83(1). p. 238–244.

[4] Grimsby, O. and Rivard, J. Science, theory and clinical application in orthopaedic manual physical therapy: Scientific therapeutic exercise progressions (STEP): The neck and upper extremity. The Academy of Graduate Physical Therapy, Inc. 2009, 275.

[5] Because of their location, some authors assert that the lateral pterygoids can be palpated intraorally. (See: Tuerp, J.C. and Minagi, S. (2001) Palpation of the lateral pterygoid region in TMD: Where is the evidence? *Journal of Dentistry.* 29(7). p. 475–483, and Stratmann, U. et al. (2000) Clinical anatomy and palpability of the inferior lateral pterygoid muscle. *Journal of Prosthetic*

Dentistry. 83(5). p. 548–554). A more recent study (Stelzenmüller, W., Weber, N.-I., Özkan, V. et al. (2006) Is the lateral pterygoid muscle palpable? A pilot study for determining the possibilities of palpating the lateral pterygoid muscle. *International Poster, Journal of Dentistry and Oral Medicine. 8(1) Poster 301,* employing MRI and electromyogram verification, concluded that the lateral pterygoid's "muscle structure and pain sensation can be determined by digital palpation and subsequently treated by functional massage." This outcome is consistent with our clinical experience that addressing this area is an effective approach to alleviating TMD symptoms. (Thanks to Dr. Leon Chaitow for these references.)

[6] Lippold, C., Danesh, G., Schilgen, M., Derup, B., and Hackenberg, L. (2006) Relationship between thoracic, lordotic, and pelvic inclination and craniofacial morphology in adults. *The Angle Orthodontist.* 76. p. 779–785.

[7] Rocabado Seaton, M. and Iglarsh, Z.A. (1990) *The Musculoskeletal Approach to Maxillofacial Pain.* Lippincott Williams & Wilkins.

[8] Cuccia, A. and Caradonna, C. (2009) The relationship between the stomatognathic system and body posture. *Clinics.* 64(1). p. 61–66.

Picture credits

Figures 15.1, 15.2, 15.5, 15.6, 15.7, and 15.8 courtesy of Primal Pictures, used by permission.

Figures 15.3, 15.4, 15.9, 15.10, 15.11, and 15.12 courtesy of Advanced-Trainings.com.

Study Guide

The Pterygoids

1 **How can you distinguish the medial pterygoid from other nearby structures?**

a press gently but firmly on the medial mandible and wait for change
b ask the client to make small, slow jaw movements
c glands will be softer than the muscle attachment
d glands will be firmer than the muscle attachment

2 **What is the intention of the Medial Pterygoid Technique?**

a coordinate bilateral condyle movement upon jaw depression
b coordinate bilateral condyle movement upon jaw retraction
c greater muscle tone, lowered myofascial adaptability, and bilateral coordination
d greater myofascial adaptability, lowered muscle tone, and bilateral coordination

3 **What is the action of the lateral pterygoids on the TMJ?**

a initiate jaw elevation by pulling jaw superiorly and disc anteriorly
b initiate jaw depression by pulling jaw and discs anteriorly
c initiate jaw depression by pulling mandibular condyles inferiorly and discs anteriorly
d initiate jaw elevation by pulling jaw superiorly and disc posteriorly

4 **What is the practitioner feeling for in assessment phase of the Lateral Pterygoid Technique?**

a the client's ability to open the jaw completely
b which mandibular condyle moves later upon opening, indicating the tighter lateral pterygoid
c the client's ability to shift the jaw laterally
d which mandibular condyle moves first upon opening, indicating the tighter lateral pterygoid

5 **What is the stated purpose of the Lateral Pterygoid Technique?**

a increase range of jaw depression
b increase myofascial differentiation and elasticity
c reduce and balance resting tone by refining proprioception
d increase range of jaw protrusion

For Answer Keys, visit www.Advanced-Trainings.com/v2key/

The Masseter, Part II

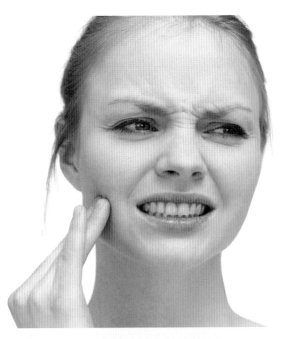

Figure 16.1

The masseter is a common site of jaw pain, and myofascial tension here can be involved in temporomandibular joint disorders, jaw pain, teeth grinding, headaches, whiplash pain, breathing and sleep disturbances, and more.

The masseter bites, chews, and clenches. It is active in talking, in neck stabilization, and whenever your jaw isn't hanging open. When it is overly active or tight, the masseter can play a key role in temporomandibular joint disorders (TMJD), jaw pain, teeth grinding, headaches, whiplash pain, breathing and sleep disturbances, and more. Since touching and pressing one's own masseter is an instinctual response to jaw pain or tightness (Figure 16.1), can skilled touch help relieve any of the many conditions related to the masseter?

I'll address this question, but first, let's review some interesting masseter facts. The word "masseter" is from the Greek μασᾶσθαι (masasthai, "to chew"). The word "massage" is thought to arise from a similar but distinct Greek verb, μάσσω (massō, "to handle, touch, to work with the hands, to knead dough"). Attaching to the zygomatic bone (cheekbone), the masseter inserts at the rear of the mandible (jawbone), where it exerts to elevate (raise) the mandible.

The masseter is sometimes said to be the strongest muscle in the body. This is probably true, at least in terms of the amount of pressure it produces. (The soleus typically pulls strongest overall; the gluteus maximus is the bulkiest; and the heart, eye, and tongue muscles are the most active.) With all muscles of the jaw working together, the masseter can close the teeth with forces as strong as 55 pounds on the incisors, or 200 pounds on the molars. And, according to the *Guinness Book of Records*, in 1986 Richard Hofmann of Lake City, Florida achieved a bite strength of 975 pounds for two full seconds.

The masseter achieves its extraordinary pressure though its leverage on the mandible, and the fulcrum for this tremendous leverage are the two relatively small temporomandibular

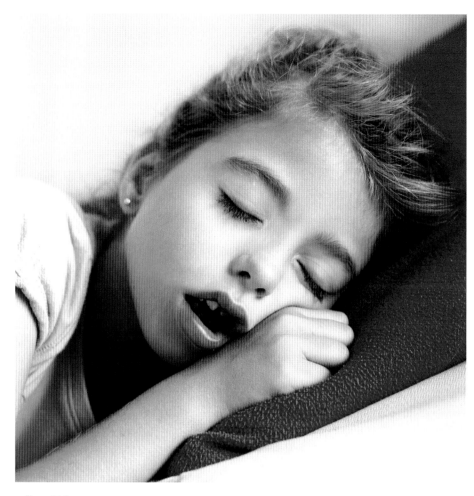

Figure 16.2

The masseter is active whenever our jaw is closed, relaxing only when we sleep or let our mouth open.

joints (TMJs). When the bite forces are aligned and balanced across the left and right TMJs, the articular discs provide the slip and glide these joints need in order to move, even while under incredible compression (see Chapter 14, *The Masseter, Temporalis, and Digastrics,* Figures 14.5 and 14.6). When the forces of the masseters and jaw muscles are not aligned, or balanced, they can squeeze, bind, or irritate the joint, leading to TMJ pain. (Chapter 14 introduces ways to assess and work with the masseter's role in jaw alignment issues, but the two additional masseter techniques in this chapter can also be applied to alignment issues.)

The masseter gets it strength from its complex "multipennate" arrangement—its layered muscle fibers converge diagonally on several internal tendons, analogous to a three-dimensional, many-layered feather with multiple shafts. This arrangement allows many muscle fibers to attach to each tendon, making it a powerful "low gear" muscle, with extra-strong pull over a short distance.

Besides being anatomically configured for high strength and leverage, the masseter has some of the highest resting tone in the body. This is related to two facts:

1. When we are upright, the jaw is held closed mostly by muscular tone (i.e. tension) in the masseters, along with the temporalis and medial pterygoids. Since we are usually upright when we are awake, the jaw muscles are working a very high percentage of the time, resting only when we sleep or allow our mouths to open (Figure 16.2).

2. Neurologically, this high level of resting tone self-perpetuates by keeping the masseters on near-constant alert. The low level of tension in the masseter continuously stimulates the muscle spindles within the belly of the masseter, reinforcing a constant, low-level stretch reflex, like the one tested when the patellar

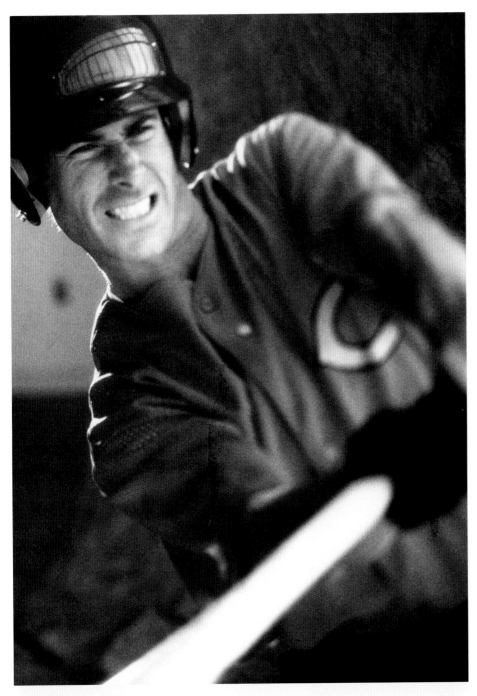

Figure 16.3
The masseter is active whenever the mandible needs stabilization, such as in jumping, impacts, or other activities (such as batting) that might knock the teeth together.

tendon is tapped with a reflex hammer. And like a patellar ligament tap, this reflex loop makes the masseter reactive and fast-acting, helping it adapt and adjust quickly during the motions of chewing, talking, and biting—and in its role as a stabilizer of the mandible and anterior neck (Figure 16.3).

Of course, a tense and reactive masseter has drawbacks. Tension here can be a contributor to TMJ pain, headaches, sleep disturbances, bruxism (teeth grinding), and other conditions. And the masseter itself can often be a primary source of pain. Although there is debate about the exact mechanism that causes myofascial trigger points, the masseter ranks as either the most common, or the second most common, of all the places where these painful myofascial points appear.

Does too much coffee make you grit your teeth? In-vitro experiments have shown that masseter muscle cells are chemically more sensitive to caffeine than other muscles in the body, due to their high resting tone and low reactivity threshold. Caffeine intake (as well as nicotine, alcohol, surgical anesthetics, and other drugs) has been observed to increase masseter tonus and/or worsen TMJ symptoms.

So far, we've listed anatomical, functional, neurological, and chemical causes of masseter tension. As if those aren't enough, there are also clear body-mind dimensions of jaw tightness as well. Although the clichéd formula of "jaw tension = anger" is sometimes derided as an over-simplification of the nuanced and highly individualized ways that emotions are reflected in the body, even mainstream medical literature commonly cites stress, anxiety, and anger as significant contributors to jaw tension, bruxism, and TMJ problems. For example, the Mayo Clinic lists "anxiety, stress, tension, anger, frustration and an aggressive or competitive personality type" amongst the causes of bruxism.

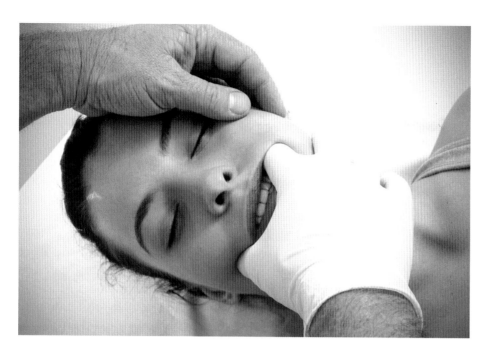

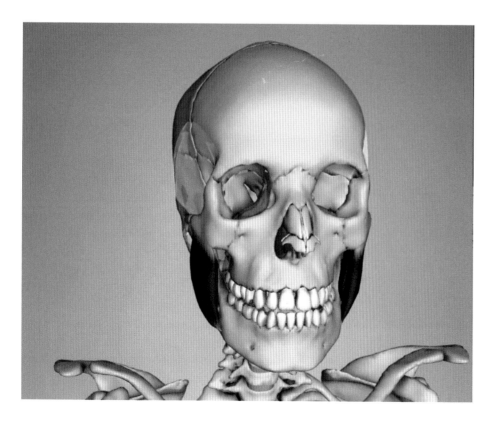

So, can hands-on work help? Skilled manual therapy can modulate masseter tension and resulting conditions in at least three ways:

1. By gently increasing myofascial differentiation and elasticity within the muscle itself.
2. By reducing the level of resting tone, via the relaxation caused by direct pressure and massaging of muscles; and by stimulation of Golgi tendon reflexes which help balance muscle-spindle reactivity.
3. By reducing overall stress and sympathetic nervous system activation.

To help you apply this information, I'll describe two masseter techniques that may appear simple at first glance. If they already seem familiar to you, take a moment to look for a new or forgotten aspect. Each of these techniques has subtlety and detail that may, at first, not be apparent.

Masseter Technique (Intraoral)

There are many ways to work with the masseter from outside the mouth (for example, see Chapter 14). But working intraorally (inside the mouth) allows access to different parts of the masseter and surrounding tissues, especially its tendinous attachments on the mandible and zygomatic arch, where Golgi tendon organs are concentrated.

When using this technique, all the customary considerations about intraoral work apply. Be sure to explain the purpose for working this way to your client, and get explicit permission first. Practice sanitary procedures like glove disposal and hand washing; ask about latex allergies; and be familiar with any local scope-of-practice stipulations (some US states require specific training or endorsement to be qualified to work within the mouth, and a small minority prohibit it outright).

As mentioned in Chapter 15, keep in mind that the mouth is the only place where we work that

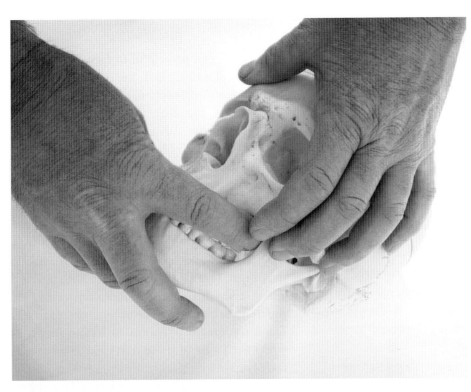

Figures 16.4/16.5/16.6

In the Masseter Technique (Intraoral), the masseter is worked between the forefinger of the gloved hand and the fingertips of the outside hand. Active client movements include jaw clenching and releasing.

is even more sensitive than your hands—your clients are feeling you even more acutely than you're feeling them. Move slowly, deliberately, gently. Find a comfortable, supported stance that allows you to keep your own neck, back, shoulders, and arms relaxed.

Typically, apply this technique on the opposite side of the client's body from where you're standing—in other words, when standing on your client's right, use your right hand to work intraorally on his or her left masseter (Figure 16.4). This allows the curve of your hand to better fit the shape of your client's jaw, and avoids the "fishhook" effect of pulling the mouth open when working the same side.

Gently slide your forefinger along the top teeth, back into the cavity between the teeth and the masseter muscle (Figure 16.5 and 16.6). Your finger pad will be against the teeth, and the nail side will be against the medial side (inside) of the masseter. Ask you client to firmly clench his or her teeth together. If you're in the right place, this will squeeze your finger between the masseter and the teeth. Try it on yourself now—this is the best way to understand the placement and active participation needed.

Once you're in position with your forefinger, use the fingertips of your outer hand to press the masseter against the inside finger. Gently roll the inside finger to feel for tissue restrictions within the masseter itself. When you find a denser area, wait for it to soften. Your client can clench and unclench to aid this process. Work along the masseter's length and width, paying special attention to the muscle's attachments: superiorly, up under the zygomatic arch (be gentle, as a branch of the trigeminal nerve exits the skull here), and inferiorly on the lateral mandible. Gently press into these attachments and wait for the overall reduction in muscle tone that signals a Golgi tendon organ-induced shift in resting tone. Repeat on the other side.

Since the masseter's angle gives it a small amount of lateral pull, this technique will be indicated when you see the jaw pull to one side upon opening. In this case, you'd typically work the masseter and temporalis on the same side as the jaw pulls towards, and then recheck. (For other contributors to jaw alignment, see Chapters 14 and 15.)

See video of the
Masseter (Intraoral)
Technique at
www.a-t.tv/tb03

Key points: Masseter Technique (Intraoral)

Indications include:
- Masseter tension, especially when accompanied by temporomandibular joint disorders (TMJD), jaw pain, bruxism, headaches, whiplash pain, breathing or sleep disturbances. Same-side lateral deviation of jaw.

Purpose
- Increase differentiation and myofascial elasticity of the masseter.
- Reduce any excessive resting tone of the masseter.
- Reduce overall stress and sympathetic nervous system activation.

Instructions
After obtaining explicit permission from the client for intraoral work:
1. Standing on the opposite side of the masseter you're addressing, slide your forefinger between the masseter and the upper teeth, with the nail side of the finger against the medial masseter.
2. Ask your client to "clench your teeth, hard." This will help confirm that you are in between the masseter and the upper teeth, and will work the medial aspect of the masseter.
3. Feel for areas of tissue density and inelasticity within the masseter, working it between your outer fingers and the inner one.

Movements
- Active and forceful jaw elevation (clenching the teeth).

Mandibular Fascia Technique

Although it can be helpful to focus on one side of the jaw at a time, as in the intraoral Masseter Technique above, functionally, the jaw's two sides always work together. The Mandibular Fascia Technique (from Advanced-Trainings.com lead instructor Larry Koliha) is a great option for finishing and balancing your jaw work with the masseter, since it addresses both sides simultaneously.

Begin by using the palms and thenar eminences of both hands (Figure 16.7) to feel into just the outer layers of skin and superficial fascia over the masseters and jaw (Figure 16.8). Use a gentle downward (caudal or inferior) pressure to sense and release any tissue restrictions or side-to-side differences; but just in the outer layers of tissue. Don't use cream or lotion, at least not yet, as you'll need a bit of friction to feel these superficial layers—with a lubricant, you may be working the muscles themselves, but you'll be sliding over the outer fascial layers, which are an important part of the jaw's structural makeup.

Once the outermost layers feel differentiated, elastic, and even from side-to-side, repeat this technique, but engage a slightly deeper tissue layer each time. With practice and sensitivity, you can often feel and work each of these layers in turn:

1. The skin and sub-dermal layers (which have varying amount of adipose cells within them);
2. The parotid fascia (a continuation of the chest and neck fascia (Figure 16.9) associated with the platysma muscle, which contains its own muscle fibers parallel to the masseter (Figure 16.8);
3. Posteriorly, the parotid glands and ducts that the parotid fascia surrounds (gentle pressure here is usually well-tolerated);
4. The masseter muscles, which themselves have two or three layers (depending on which anatomy text you consult), with the outer layer usually the most textured and tendinous, and the inner layer the softest and most muscular;

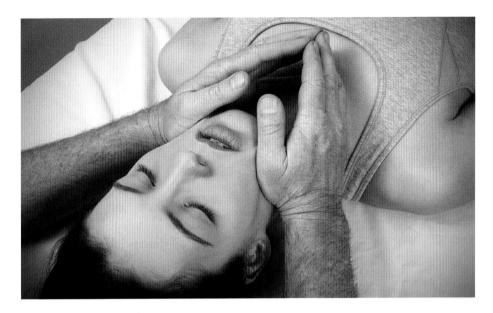

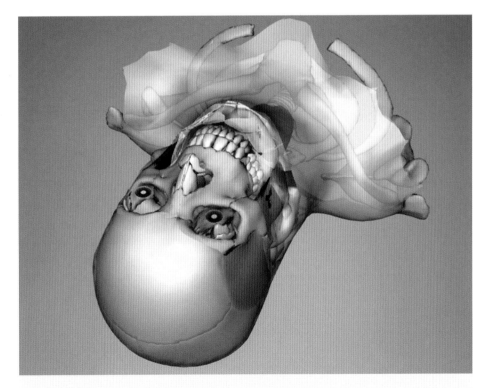

Figures 16.7/16.8

The Mandibular Fascia Technique can bring closure to a jaw session. Address each tissue layer in turn, from the superficial and deep cervical fasciae, to the jaw's parotid and buccopharyngeal fasciae, keeping in mind their continuity with the fasciae of the head and torso.

5. Deep and anterior to the masseters, the deeper mucosal layers of the mouth cavity;
6. And finally, the teeth, gums, and bones of the upper and lower jaw.

Once you've slowly worked down to the level you want, you'll be passively depressing (opening) the jaw with your slow, sliding movement. If you

---

Key points: Mandibular Fascia Technique

Indications include:
- Masseter tension, especially when accompanied by temporomandibular joint disorders (TMJD), jaw pain, bruxism, headaches, whiplash pain, breathing or sleep disturbances.
- Same-side lateral deviation of jaw.
- Preparation (before) or integration (after) intraoral or deeper jaw work.

Purpose
- Differentiate fascial layers related to jaw depression and elevation.
- Balance asymmetrical movements (lateral deviation) of the TMJ.
- Reduce any excessive resting tone of the masseter.
- Reduce overall stress and sympathetic nervous system activation.
- Bring closure and a sense of balance after other jaw work.

Instructions
1. Using the palms or thenar eminences bilaterally, gently apply caudal (inferior) pressure to the superficial fascia of the mandible (over the masseter).
2. Feel for and gently release any tissue restrictions or side-to-side differences.
3. Repeat, working subsequent layers of fascia.

Movements
- Work with pace, pressure, and communication so that the client can allow passive jaw depression (opening) and easy, relaxed breathing.

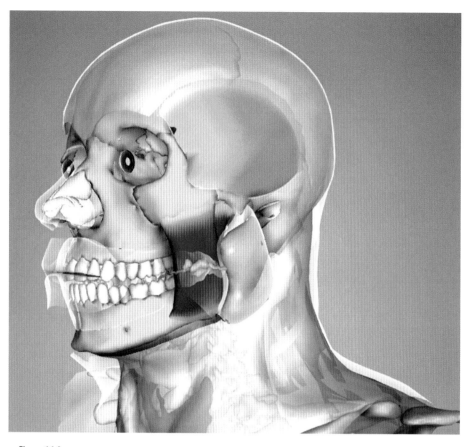

Figure 16.9

The parotid fascia (green) surrounds the parotid glands, has embedded muscle cells, and is contiguous with the superficial fascia of the neck and chest associated with the platysma.

feel your client resist this opening, slow down, come back out a layer, ask for breath, and wait for the masseters to let go.

A variation: in our trainings, we sometimes encounter manual therapists who were trained never to apply downward (caudal) pressure to the face, for fear of accelerating the tissue sag of aging. If this is a concern, an alternative to the downward pressure described above would be to apply gentle upward (cephalad) pressure instead, as the client slowly opens the jaw. This is similar to the Masseter and Temporalis Technique in Chapter 14, but instead applied here to the facial layers listed above.

Of course, masseter issues do not exist in isolation. The jaw, being very mobile and suspended primarily by soft tissue, is particularly vulnerable to imbalance and strain elsewhere in the body. For example, jaw tension is one response to the instability of a whiplash injury to the neck, as the masseter, temporalis, and other jaw muscles attempt to brace and stabilize the injured area by immobilizing the mandible (which is an attachment site for the hyoids, platysma, and superficial fascia of the neck).

As always, when working with TMJ pain, be sure to also address whole-body patterns, since issues such as spinal curves, pelvis muscle tension, hip pain, pelvic angle, and posture have all been shown to correlate with jaw function. As with many other symptoms, a whole-body approach to jaw issues will yield more sustainable results and more satisfying outcomes.

References

[1] Rodrigues Corrêa, E.C. and Bérzin, F. (2004) Temporomandibular disorder and dysfunctional breathing. *Brazilian Journal of Oral Sciences.* 3(10). p. 498–502.

[2] *Guinness World Records* http://www.guinnessworldrecords.com/news/2013/4/daft-punk-track-smashes-streaming-benchmark-luis-suarez-apologises-for-bite-and-giant-mantis-robot-gets-unveiled—the-news-in-world-records-48248. [Accessed December 2015]

[3] Travell, J.G. et al. (1999) *Myofascial Pain and Dysfunction.* Williams and Wilkins. p. 330.

[4] Adnet, P.J. et al. (1996) In vitro human masseter muscle hypersensitivity: A possible explanation for increase in masseter tone. *Journal of Applied Physiology.* 80(5). p. 1547–1553.

[5] Bruxism/teeth grinding. Mayo Foundation for Medical Education and Research (MFMER), 2011. http://www.mayoclinic.com/health/bruxism/DS00337/DSECTION=causes. [Accessed December 2015]

[6] Schleip, R. (2003) Fascial plasticity: A new neurobiological explanation, Part I. *Journal of Bodywork and Movement Therapies.* 7(1). p. 14.

[7] Lippold, C. et al. (2006) Relationship between thoracic, lordotic, and pelvic inclination and craniofacial morphology in adults. *The Angle Orthodontist.* 76. p. 779–785.

[8] Fischer, M.J. et al. (2009) Influence of the temporomandibular joint on range of motion of the hip joint in patients with Complex Regional Pain Syndrome. *Journal of Manipulative and Physiological Therapeutics* (JMPT). 32 (5) p. 364–371.

[9] Cuccia, A. and Caradonna, C. (2009) The relationship between the stomatognathic system and body posture. *Clinics.* 64(1). p. 61–66.

Picture credits

Figures 16.1, 16.2, and 16.3 courtesy Thinkstock.
Figures 16.4 & 16.6, and 16.7 courtesy Advanced-Trainings.com.
Figures 16.5, 16.8, and 16.9 courtesy Primal Pictures, used by permission.

Study Guide

The Masseter, Part II

1 **In the Masseter Technique (Intraoral), why does the author recommend standing on the opposite side of the body from the side being worked?**

a to reduce danger of inadvertent biting injuries
b by standing rather than sitting you have more control over pressure used
c working across the body gives the client a sense of comfort
d the curve of your hand better matches the shape of the client's jaw

2 **According to the text, what client action in Masseter Technique (Intraoral) assists in the release?**

a retracting the jaw
b protruding the jaw
c clenching and unclenching the teeth
d laterally moving the jaw

3 **Along with the masseter, what other two muscles keep the jaw closed, according to the text?**

a temporalis and medial pterygoid
b temporalis and lateral pterygoid
c digastric and temporalis
d medial and lateral pterygoids

4 **All of the following could be said to be valid reasons to work elsewhere in the body when addressing TMJ issues. Which one is mentioned in the text?**

a working too long on the TMJ can aggravate pain or dysfunction
b the TMJ is affected by posture and whole-body relationships
c working elsewhere helps the client not fixate on the pain in their jaw
d working elsewhere encourages a parasympathetic response, which helps relax the jaw muscles

5 **According to the text, what is one reason the masseter has a high resting tone?**

a most people don't want to appear slack-jawed
b we are an angry, aggressive culture (evidenced by lower masseter tension in other societies)
c the masseter holds the mouth closed while upright
d the patellar-mandibular reflex increases tone in muscle spindles

For Answer Keys, visit www.Advanced-Trainings.com/v2key/

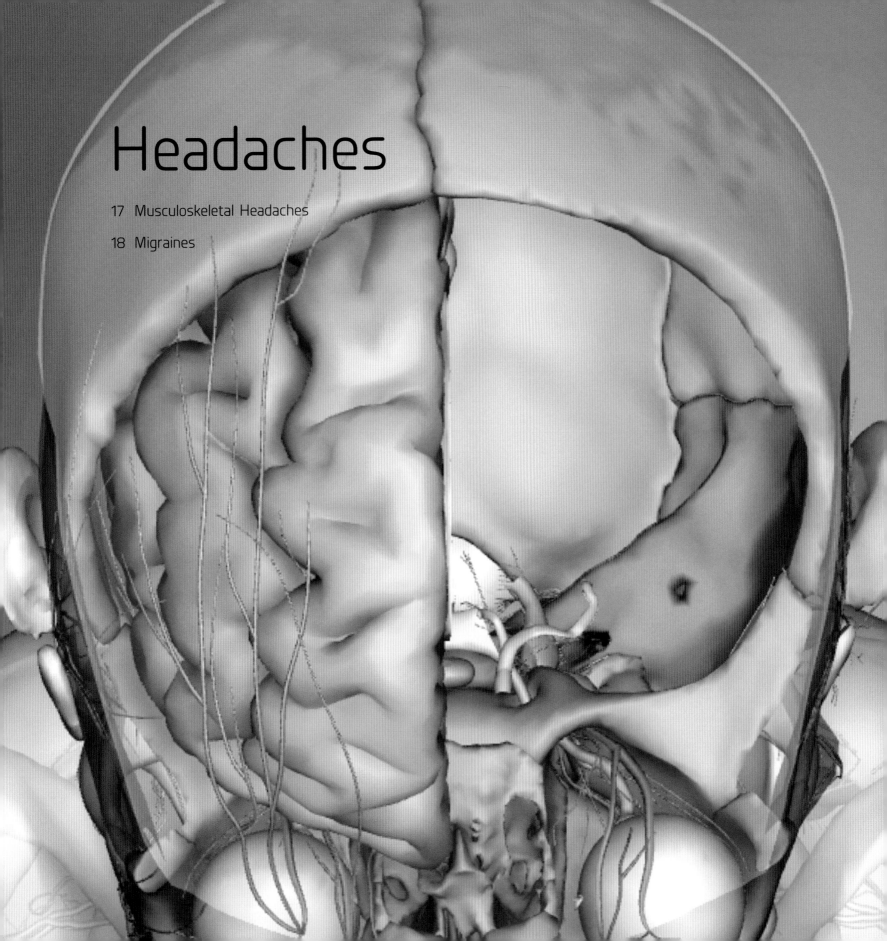

Headaches

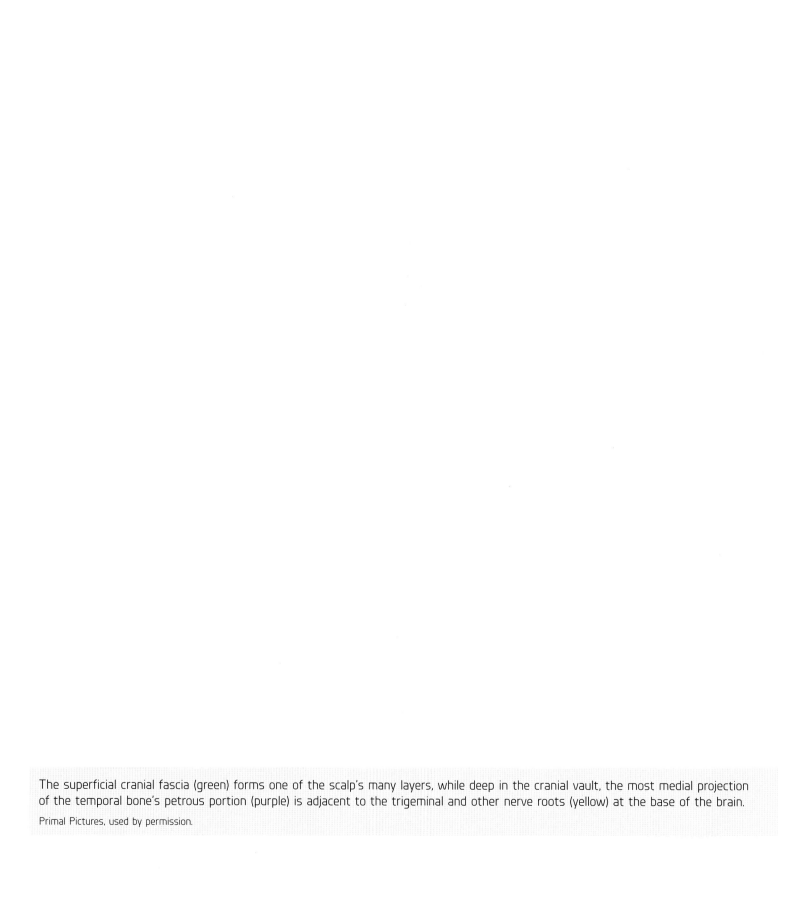

The superficial cranial fascia (green) forms one of the scalp's many layers, while deep in the cranial vault, the most medial projection of the temporal bone's petrous portion (purple) is adjacent to the trigeminal and other nerve roots (yellow) at the base of the brain.

Take a guess: how many kinds of headaches are there? With Google and a few minutes, you can compile a list of hundreds of distinct types of headache, including: cryogenic headache (after eating ice cream), hair wash headache (found most commonly in Indian women whose hair, due to its length, is wet from washing a good proportion of the time, and thus heavy), coital cephalalgia (or "morning after" headache), ictal headache (accompanying seizures), thunderclap headache (sudden, severe onset), and many, many more. How would you begin to formulate a coherent approach to dealing with headaches when there are so many categories, kinds, and causes?

Fortunately, we can narrow it down. Headaches are conventionally classified as either *primary* (not caused by another condition) or *secondary* (caused by another condition). Examples of secondary headaches include those resulting from head injuries, from metabolic and medical conditions, etc. Although hands-on work can help in many cases, for these and other types of secondary headaches, referral to a physician first is usually advisable. This is generally a good practice with any persistent or recurring headache.[1]

Primary headaches (those not caused by another condition) can be further sub-classified as arising from:

1. *Musculoskeletal* origins (such as tension-type headaches and others related to myofascial or articular restriction);
2. *Neurological and neurovascular* factors (such as in migraines and cluster headaches); or
3. *Commingled* causes (that is, arising from a combination of musculoskeletal and neurological sources).

	Musculoskeletal Headaches	Migraine Headaches
Pain location	Typically bilateral	Typically one-sided
Common pain descriptors	"Pressure" or "squeezing"	"Throbbing" or "stabbing"
Response to activity	Usually no change[2]	Usually worsened
Sensory Epiphenomena	Not commonly associated with nausea, light/sound sensitivity, or aura (unless commingled)	Consistently accompanied by either nausea, light/sound sensitivity, or aura (visual disturbances)
Hands-on goal	Reduce myofascial tension and hypersensitivity	Reduce cranial compression

Table 17.1 Comparison of musculoskeletal (or tension-type) headaches and migraines (or neurovascular type headaches). Commingled headaches, since they arise from both musculoskeletal and neurovascular causes, can have characteristics of both types.

1 The importance of referring persistent headaches to a physician for evaluation was driven home to me several years ago when our office manager at Advanced-Trainings was diagnosed with a brain tumor that eventually, and tragically, proved fatal. Recurrent headaches had been her only symptom. Don't alarm your clients of course, but do insist on screening for recurring, severe, or persistent headaches.
2 Although migraine pain is typically aggravated by activity or movement (climbing stairs, bending over, etc.), cluster headaches (also a neurovascular headache) can sometimes be relieved by vigorous aerobic activity.

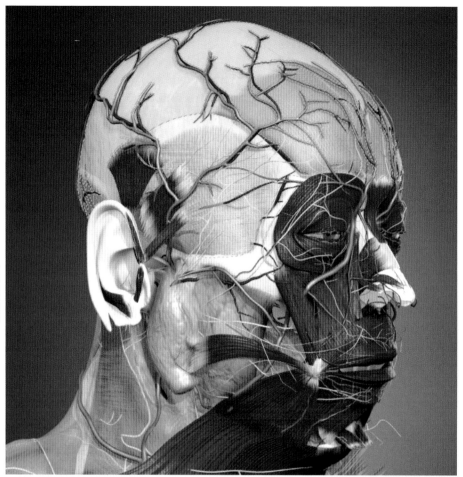

See video of the Galea Aponeurotica Technique at www.a-t.tv/hc05

Figure 17.1

The superficial fascia of the cranium (dark green) is a tough fibro-adipose layer just under the skin: the galea aponeurosis (light green) is deep to the superficial fascia, and is the fascial portion of the frontalis and occipitalis muscles. These layers play a role in many tension and musculoskeletal headaches.

Musculoskeletal or tension-type headaches are by far the most common kind of headache, even if not necessarily the most severe. Hands-on manual therapy can help, for both mild and severe forms. A recent systematic review of manual therapy randomized controlled trials concluded that hands-on work can reduce both the frequency and the intensity of chronic tension-type headaches. In this, the first of two chapters on headaches, I'll describe two techniques that are effective for this category of headache. In Chapter 18, we'll focus on ways to help mitigate migraines and neurovascular headaches.

Galea Aponeurotica Technique

The superficial fascia of the scalp (Figures 17.1 and 17.2) is directly continuous with the superficial fascial membranes of the back of the neck, and by extension, the superficial fascia of the rest of the body. Its position on the crown of the head gives it the unique role of connecting the front of the body to the back, and left side to right. As such, it is a mediator and transmitter of fascial stresses and compensations elsewhere in the body. Also known as the subcutaneous fibro-adipose layer, it lies between the outer layers of skin and the underlying galea aponeurotica or epicranium. Although this deeper layer is also mainly membranous, it contains the muscle fibers of the occipitofrontalis muscles. Because the galea is continuous laterally with the temporal fascia overlying the temporalis muscle, it is particularly sensitive to jaw tension. Deep to the galea is the pericranium on the bones of the skull themselves (Figure 17.2).

Besides transmitting strain and referred pain from the rest of the body's fasciae, the cranial layers can play a direct role in headaches associated with face, neck, and eye-strain, as well as mental exertion or stress. The adaptability and pliability of these layers is essential to free motion of the underlying sutures and cranial bones. Suture restrictions can play a role in both musculoskeletal and migraine headaches, and so ensuring the cranial fasciae's differentiation and freedom is a logical first step in working with headaches.

Interestingly, the scalp is also one of the areas of the body that has specialized nerve fibers (C-tactile afferents) which are thought to play a role in the brain's "positive" (pleasant, calming, or socially affiliative) emotional responses to touch. Since headaches of all kinds are often accompanied by upset, stress, or emotional disquiet, it is useful to keep in mind that hands-on work with the scalp can have particularly comforting body-mind effects.

To release the cranial fasciae, use your fingertips to move the various layers against each other, and against the skull. We're not scrubbing the surface of the scalp or shampooing the hair; we're sliding, shearing, and freeing the fascial layers themselves. Imagine loosening the rind of a cantaloupe around the flesh of the melon: use firm, deep transverse pressure to assess and release adhesions, pulls, and thickenings. Use a decisive but sensitive touch; be patient and thorough. Spend several minutes with this technique, working the various layers over the entire head, adding client's active movements of the eyes, face, and eyebrows once the outer layers have been differentiated (Figures 17.3–17.7).

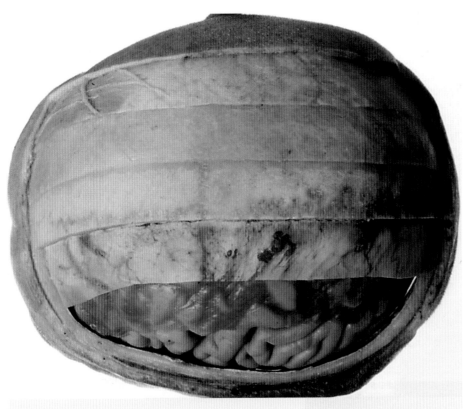

Figure 17.2

A stepped dissection of the cranial fascial layers. From bottom to top, the visible layers include the arachnoid mater (thin, red layer just superficial to the brain); the dura mater; the bony cranium; pericranium; galea aponeurotica (with the muscle fibers of frontalis and occipitalis visible anteriorly and posteriorly); and the superficial fascia of the scalp (continuous with the skin, and forming the outer layer in this view).

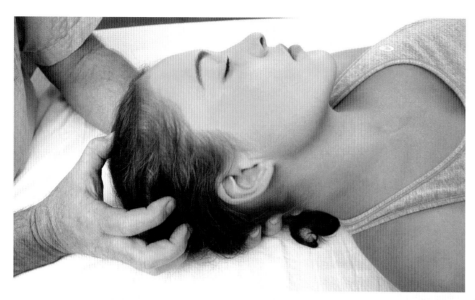

Figure 17.3

Use firm finger pressure to slide the superficial and deep fasciae of the scalp against one another, and against the bones of the cranium. Pay particular attention to any thickenings over the slightly raised lines of the sutures.

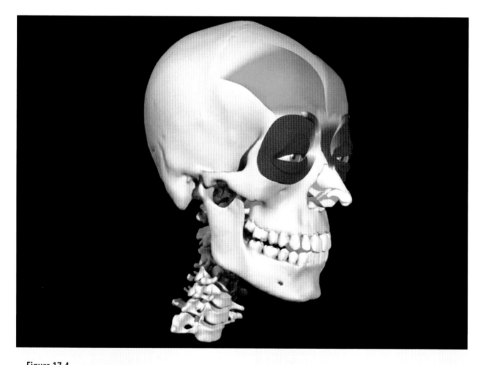

Figure 17.4

The muscle fibers of the frontalis muscles (in green).

Key points: Superficial and Deep Fascia of the Scalp Technique

Indications include:
- Tension and neurovascular headaches.

Purpose
- Increase differentiation (sliding and shearing) of the cranial fascia layers.
- Increase options for mobility of the underlying cranial sutures.
- ANS calming via stimulation of C-tactile afferent nerve fibers.

Instructions
1. Use deep transverse pressure to move (shear) the cranial fascial layers against each other and against the skull, paying attention to adhesions, pulls, thickenings, and restricted areas.
2. Once the outer fascial layers have been mobilized, ask client to experiment with active movements, focusing on those that relieve headache pain or mobility restriction.

Movements
- Exaggerated movement of the eyes, jaw, face, and eyebrows.

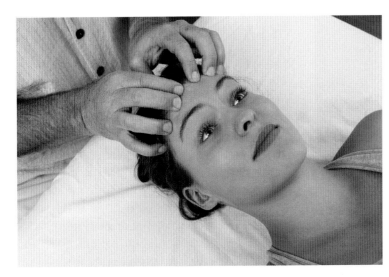

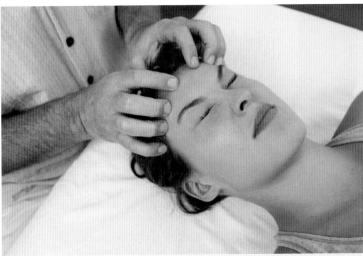

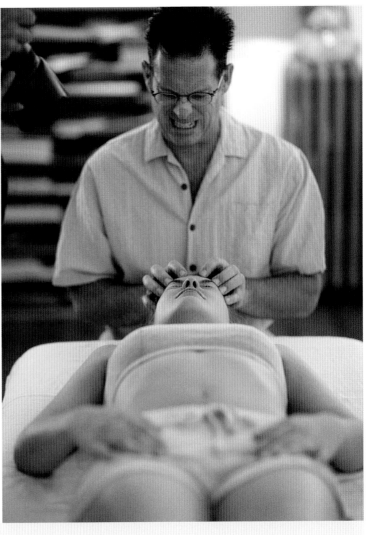

Figures 17.5/17.6/17.7

Because the galea aponeurotica contains the muscle fibers of frontalis and occipitalis, engaging your client's active and exaggerated eye, brow, and face movements will deepen and extend the fascial release. (And no, it isn't necessary to work so hard that you grit your own teeth, but it can be helpful to show your client the faces you'd like her to make.)

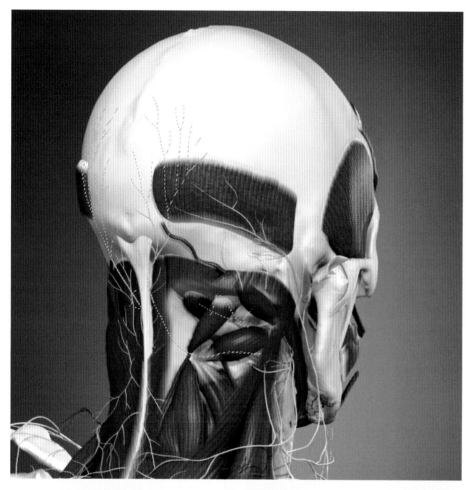

Figure 17.8

The central nuchal ligament (orange) and the suboccipital and greater occipital nerves (green), which pass through the suboccipital muscles and can play a role in tension-type headaches of the posterior head.

Nuchal Window Technique

Neck pain correlates with tension-type headaches, migraines, and commingled types. Working the sub-occipital muscles is a well-known way to relieve tension-type headaches. The Nuchal Window Technique is a variation on this approach. With your client supine, place your fingertips longitudinally along either side of the nuchal ligament, with your middle fingers just under the occipital ridge at the superior end of the nuchal ligament (Figures 17.9 and 17.10). With firm but patient pressure, encourage the musculature and soft tissue on either side of the ligament to release laterally. Our intention is to "open the window" of the suboccipital space in order to give more room to the small muscles there, and the important cervical nerves that pass between them (Figure 17.8), often a source of posterior head pain. Although very effective for tension-type headaches, working the suboccipital region has sometimes been observed to worsen migraine headaches, perhaps because it may increase cranial circulation. Review the distinctions in Table 17.1, and if you suspect migraine elements, use suboccipital work carefully, while watching how your client responds.

Musculoskeletal headaches are seldom related to just the cranial fascia or suboccipital muscles: jaw, neck, eye, and shoulder tension will also contribute to many headache patterns, so think broadly. It is worth remembering that like all pain, headache pain is a perception, and as such, is influenced by many factors in addition to the physical properties of the tissues involved. For example, generalized pain hypersensitivity (or hyperalgesia) has been correlated with chronic tension-type headaches, which suggests that pain processing in the central nervous system plays an important role in this type of headache. As with pain elsewhere, the sensations triggered by skilled touch can be effective in changing pain perception and pain

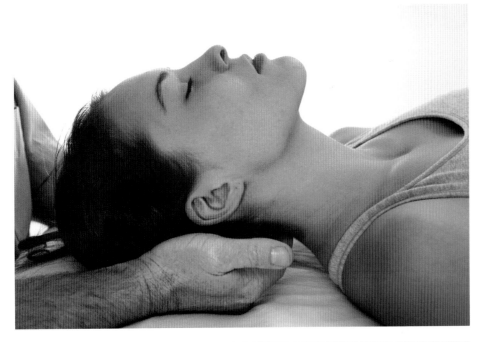

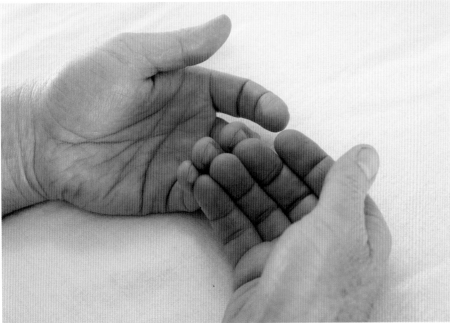

Figures 17.9/17.10

In the Nuchal Window Technique, your fingers encourage lateral differentiation of the myofascia on either side of the longitudinal nuchal ligament, opening the "window" of the suboccipital space.

processing patterns. With headaches in particular, we are working with much more than just the physical tissues involved.

Although headaches have many dimensions and causes, the two techniques described in this chapter are simple but extremely effective hands-on tools that will provide relief and help to prevent recurrence when there is musculoskeletal involvement in headache pain. In the next chapter, we'll look at ways to address migraine headaches, adding more options to your technique toolbox.

> **Key points:** Nuchal Window Technique
>
> **Indications include:**
> - Tension headaches, especially those with posterior head pain.
>
> **Purpose**
> - Increase layer differentiation to create space, "open the window" for the suboccipital muscles and the nerves which pass through this area.
>
> **Instructions**
> 1. With a firm touch, gently and patiently encourage the myofascia on either side of the nuchal ligament to release laterally.
> 2. Wait for response; reposition elsewhere along nuchal ligament; repeat.

References

[1] Robbins, M.S. and Lipton, R.B. (2010) The epidemiology of primary headache disorders. *Seminars in Neurology*. 30. p. 107–119.

[2] Chaibi, A. and Russell, M.B. (2014) Manual therapies for primary chronic headaches: A systematic review of randomized controlled trials. *The Journal of Headache and Pain*. 15(1). p. 67.

[3] McGlone, F., Wessberg, J., and Olausson, H. (2014) Discriminative and affective touch: Sensing and feeling. *Neuron*. 82(4). p. 737–755.

[4] Ashina, S., Bendtsen, L., Lyngberg, A.C., Lipton, R.B., Hajiyeva, N., and Jensen, R. (2015) Prevalence of neck pain in migraine and tension-type headache: A population study. *Cephalalgia*. 35(3) p. 211–219.

[5] Pielsticker, A., Haag, G., Zaudig, M., and Lautenbacher, S. (2005) Impairment of pain inhibition in chronic tension-type headache. *Pain*. 118(1–2). p. 215–223.

Picture credits

Figures 17.1, 17.2, 17.4, and 17.8 courtesy Primal Pictures, used by permission.
Figures 17.3, 17.5, 17.6. 17.7, 17.9, and 17.10 Advanced-Trainings.com.

Study Guide

Musculoskeletal Headaches

1 **The suggested strategic goal when working with migraines is to reduce:**

a suboccipital tension
b cranial compression
c jaw tension
d myofascial tension

2 **According to the text, which of these is typical of musculoskeletal headaches?**

a often bilateral
b usually one-sided
c worsens with activity
d typically nocturnal

3 **What is the stated intention when working with the cranial fascia?**

a increase proprioception
b layer differentiation
c tactile afferent nerve fiber inhibition
d stimulate circulation

4 **What does the chapter recommend for clients with persistent or reoccurring headaches?**

a lighter work
b work with caution
c deeper work
d physician referral

5 **What is the stated practitioner intention in the Nuchal Window Technique?**

a reduce cranial compression
b re-educate and release the trapezius muscles
c create space for the suboccipital muscles and nerves
d release the nuchal ligament

For Answer Keys, visit www.Advanced-Trainings.com/v2key/

Migraines

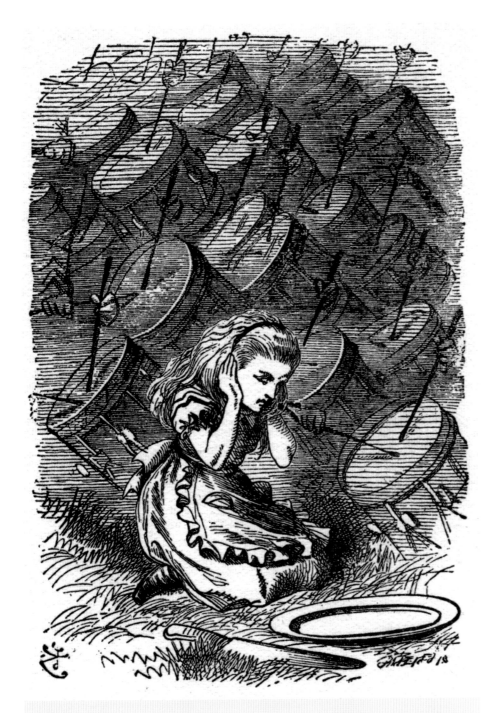

Figure 18.1

Hypersensitivity to sound and/or visual disturbances are two of the distinguishing characteristics of migraines.
An illustration by John Tenniel from Lewis Carroll's *Through the Looking Glass*. Carroll himself suffered from migraines.

What is a migraine? Good question. We don't quite know what causes migraine headaches, but we know how to recognize one. Although many people will call any severe headache a migraine, some of the distinguishing characteristics of true migraines are that they 1) tend to primarily affect one side of the head; 2) throb or pulse; 3) recur after pain-free intervals; and 4) are almost always accompanied by either nausea, photophobia (light hypersensitivity), phonophobia (sound hypersensitivity, Figure 18.1), or aura (visual disturbances, Figure 18.2) (see Table 17.1 page 175).

Migraines vary a great deal in their severity and accompanying symptoms, and are sometimes "commingled" with tension/musculoskeletal headaches. However, in the absence of a head injury or medical condition, the chances are very good that your client's headache is a true migraine if it has at least three of the four characteristics listed above. Since migraines respond differently to hands-on work than other kinds of headaches (for instance, suboccipital work often improves tension headaches, but seems to make some migraines worse), being able to distinguish migraines from musculoskeletal headaches will make your interventions more effective. (See Chapter 17 for more about recognizing musculoskeletal headaches.)

Vascular, or not?

Even though we can recognize and work with migraines, their root cause is disputed, and only partially understood. Brain tissue itself is insensitive to pain, so until relatively recently, the severe pain of migraines was thought to originate from dilation and stretching of the brain's blood vessels (Figure 18.3), which do register pain, and from the resulting pressure on the sensitive meninges and other tissues within the cranium.

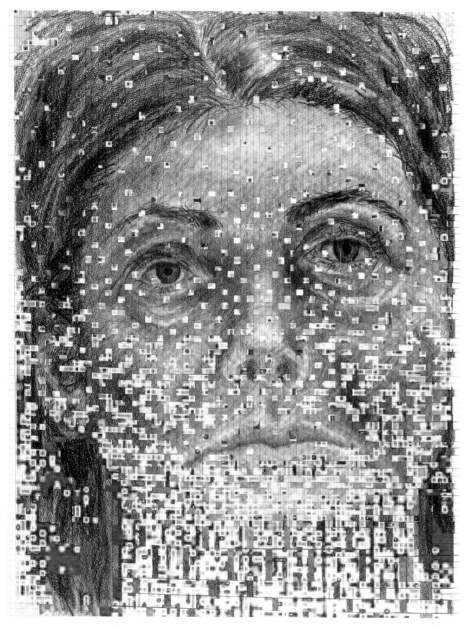

Figure 18.2

18.2: *Migraine,* Helen Donis-Keller.

Vascular dilation (vasodilation) was thought to be the cause of migraines as early as the 1700s. In more recent times, brain scans confirm that vasodilation is in fact associated with many migraines, and that this can increase blood flow up to 300 percent—but, only *before* a migraine, and only in some migraine sufferers. This same research found that during a migraine headache itself, blood circulation in the brain is normal, or even slightly reduced (1). These findings cast doubt on vasodilation as the main cause of migraines. (The results may, however, explain the observations of some migraine suffers that, if applied early enough, ice on the occiput or ice cream held on the palate can sometimes slow or stop the progression of a migraine headache, since cold is a vasoconstrictor.) Prescription drugs for migraines commonly contain vasoconstrictors, and reports are common that caffeine (also a vasoconstrictor) can help stop a migraine's progression, if used at the first sign of symptoms (although others report fewer migraines once regular caffeine use is discontinued). However, these and other remedies that rely primarily on correcting vascular dilation produce only limited success, supporting the view that there are other, non-vascular mechanisms that cause migraine pain as well.

Women get migraines more often than men, especially around times of hormonal change; up to 28 percent of all women will have migraines at some point in their lives (2). Studies of twins suggest that genetics has a 60 to 65 percent influence on the likelihood of getting migraines (3). Environmental factors have been implicated in migraines as well. Documented migraine triggers include stress, injuries, certain foods, alcohol, dehydration, physical exertion, menses and hormone fluctuations, physical or emotional stress, strong odors, flashing lights,

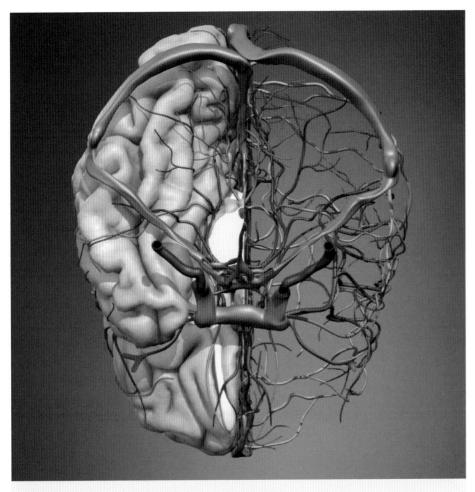

Figure 18.3

Migraines have long been classified as vascular headaches as their pain was thought to be caused by over-dilation of the veins and arteries within the cranium. Recent research suggests that the nervous system plays a much bigger role than previously thought, and that vasodilation happens only at the onset of a migraine, and only in some cases.

weather changes, allergies, sleep deprivation, hunger, fluorescent lights, tension headaches, and more (4).

Currently, the most commonly accepted view is that migraines are primarily a nervous system disorder, with a complex interplay of genetic and environmental contributors, comparable to the way that both genetics and environment contribute to conditions such as diabetes or high blood pressure. Recent research (5) suggests that migraines start as waves of nerve cell hyperactivity sweeping across the brain (Figure 18.4); the spreading waves in turn activate pain-signaling neurons in the brainstem. The root cause of these neuro-electrical "brain storms" of abnormally increased activity (known as cortical spreading depression) is unknown. The hyperactivity is followed by inhibited nerve cell excitability; the cells seem to be worn out, and this exhaustion may explain difficulty speaking or thinking clearly after migraines.

There may be other neurological factors involved as well. A study at Harvard Medical School in 2007 showed differences in migraineurs' physical brain structure. In the long-term migraine sufferers studied, the area of the somatosensory cortex corresponding to the trigeminal nerve (which supplies the head and the face, Figures 18.13–18.15) was thicker than normal (6). It is unclear whether this is a cause or an effect of migraine pain, but the authors of the study suggest that the sensory cortex's differences may help explain why some migraine sufferers also experience back pain, jaw pain, skin sensitivity, and other sensory problems along with their headaches.

Cluster headaches

Cluster headaches may be among the most painful experiences known (Figure 18.5). According to mothers who experience cluster headaches,

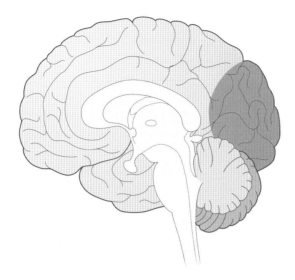

Figure 18.4

The zone affected by abnormal neuronal activity in the brain (cortical spreading depression, in red) approximately 6 minutes after the inception of a migraine headache. The size of the affected area continues to grow as the migraine progresses.

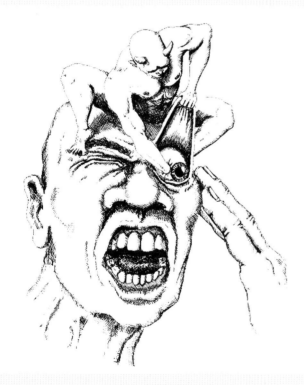

Figure 18.5

Cluster headaches involve repeating episodes of severe eye, face, or orbital pain. Like migraines, they seem to be neurological in origin. *The Cluster Headache,* JD Fletcher.

they can surpass even the pain of childbirth (7). Characterized by unilateral, sudden, and severe eye, face, or orbital pain, they can last from 15 minutes to three hours. They tend to recur in "clusters" of activity, interrupted by pain-free periods; hence their name. They are also known as "suicide headaches," due to their severity. Cluster headaches are less common than migraines, with about one-twenty-fifth the number of "clusterers" as migraineurs (8). Like migraines, cluster headaches probably have a vascular component, as dilation of cranial blood vessels is thought to put pressure on the trigeminal nerve. Also like migraines, the underlying cause of cluster headaches is unknown, but hormones, neurotransmitters, and abnormal hypothalamus activity are suspected factors.

Some cluster headaches are relieved by fresh air, or by vigorous aerobic exercise (which can worsen a migraine); increased oxygenation is the suspected mechanism (9). Probably because of trigeminal nerve involvement, hands-on work around the zygomatic arches (through the upper cheek, or intraorally), or careful but firm pressure directly on the rim of the orbit, can both be welcome first-aid measures. In terms of other hands-on techniques, cluster headaches can often be addressed like migraines, in accordance with the intentions and techniques I'll describe below.

Techniques for Migraines

Hands-on work can help migraines. Multiple studies substantiate this (10). Additionally, we see anecdotal evidence in our own private practices, and in the stories we hear from our Advanced Myofascial Techniques seminar participants.

Even though the causes and mechanisms of migraine and cluster headaches are only partially understood (as discussed in Chapter 17 and above) we've found we are often able to relieve active and acute migraines, and in many cases, it seems that we can reduce their frequency as well.

Decompressing the Head

Chapter 17 covered how tension and other musculoskeletal headaches are different from migraines (Figures 18.6 and 18.7). For common musculoskeletal (or tension-type) headaches,

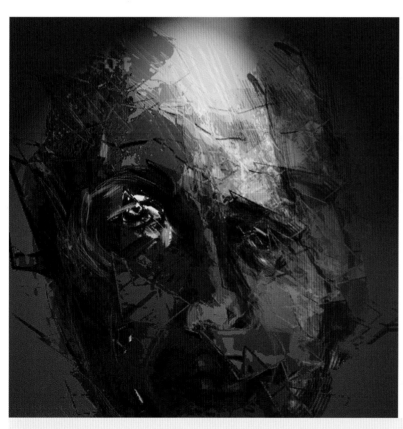

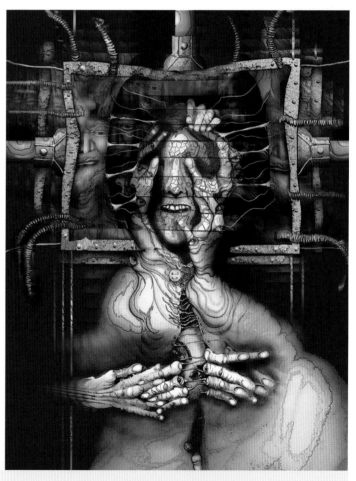

Figures 18.6/18.7

Migraines are distinguished from tension-type headaches in that they're consistently accompanied by sensory phenomena like visual disturbances (18.6, *Visual Disturbances*, Joyce Ryan), and tend to be unilateral rather than bilateral (18.7, *Overwhelm*, Rick Simpson) like musculoskeletal or tension headaches. (See Chapter 17 for more about distinguishing migraines from other headaches.)

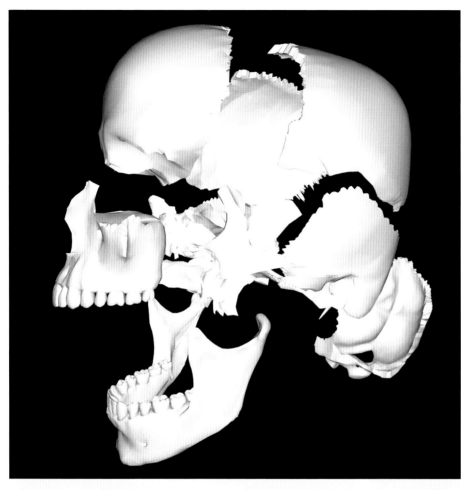

Figure 18.8

Our hands-on aim in working with migraines is to metaphorically "decompress" the bones of the cranium. The palate is one of the central keystones of the cranial structure.

See video of the Palate Technique at www.a-t.tv/nc07

our main hands-on goal is to *release any myofascial tension* contributing to the head pain. This is also a useful way to start when working with migraines, especially since many migraines are commingled with myofascial pain and restricted layer mobility, and can even be triggered by a tension headache. In the case of migraines, there is an additional step we can take. Once fascial restrictions have been released, our primary hands-on goal for working with vascular headaches becomes *reducing cranial compression*.

This empirical approach originates in my own experience as an occasional migraine sufferer. During one of my migraines, my clear sense was that relief from the crushing pain lay not in working on the outside of my head, but by getting inside my cranium itself and opening it outward from within.

I'm not able to say if "reducing cranial compression" is solely a subjective metaphor, or if the techniques described here actually diminish cranial compression in an objectively verifiable way. However, in both my personal and clinical experience, these methods reliably relieve many migraines if performed during an episode, sometimes quite dramatically. Prevention is harder to quantify, but many clients (though not all) have reported reduced headache frequency and severity when regularly performing these techniques on themselves.

Palate Technique

If our aim when working with migraines is to decompress the cranium from the inside out, what better place to get inside the head, than the palate? Not only can the hard palate be thought of as a "keystone" of the cranium's interlocking bony structure (Figure 18.8), but compression of the palate by braces or orthodontics has a known relationship with migraines and commingled headaches (11).

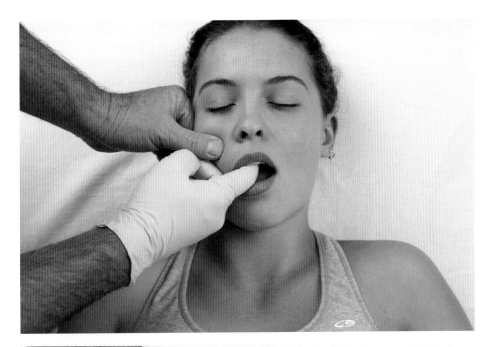

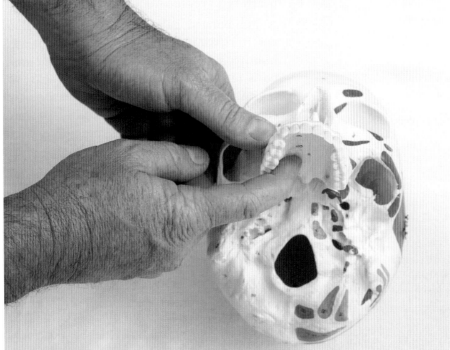

Figures 18.9/18.10

Palate Technique. Feel through the maxilla from both inside and outside the mouth. Keep your finger, hand, wrist, elbow, shoulder, and neck relaxed—any tension or discomfort in your body will markedly change your touch, and be perceived by your client.

When working the palate, all customary considerations about intraoral work apply, of course. Be sure to explain the purpose for working inside the mouth to your client and get explicit permission before you do so. Practice sanitary procedures with glove disposal and hand washing; ask about latex sensitivity; and be familiar with any local scope-of-practice stipulations (some US states require specific training or endorsement to be qualified to work within the mouth, and a small minority prohibit it outright). And mostly, keep in mind that the mouth is both personal, and very sensitive; as mentioned earlier, the inside of the mouth is the only part of the body we work that has greater touch sensitivity than our hands.

To work the palate, use your gloved index finger inside the mouth, together with the thumb of the other hand outside, feeling the maxilla and palate between your two hands (Figures 18.9 and 18.10). Use slow, static, sensitive, and firm-but-gentle pressure to feel the shape and mobility (or fixity) of the bones that make up the palate. Don't slide around with your inner finger; instead, gently and slowly press in one spot; feel for a response; and wait. Once you feel a slight drift or yielding, only then, release and move to the next spot.

Feel for unusual bony resilience (soft or hard areas, not to be mistaken for the nodules of the small glands on the posterior palate). If your client has a headache, check in (verbally and non-verbally) for feedback about any places that change the quality of the head pain. There will usually be areas where pressure will relieve or change the pain. Wait in these places with steady pressure, encouraging your client to relax, breathe, and release. Although it can take several minutes in each spot, you can often diminish the headache's intensity, and sometime relieve it completely by being patient and methodical here—"painstaking" might be just the right word.

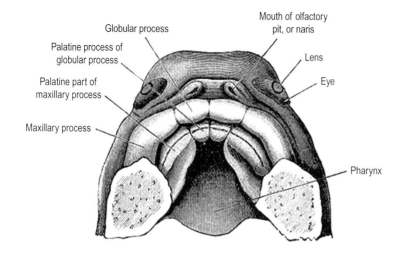

Labels: Globular process; Mouth of olfactory pit, or naris; Palatine process of globular process; Lens; Palatine part of maxillary process; Eye; Maxillary process; Pharynx

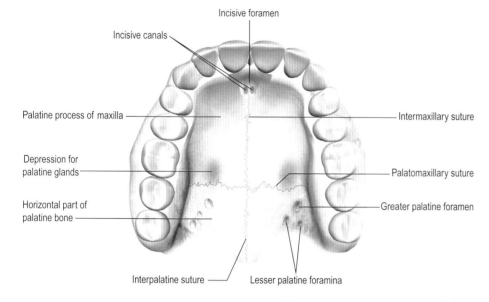

Labels: Incisive foramen; Incisive canals; Palatine process of maxilla; Intermaxillary suture; Depression for palatine glands; Palatomaxillary suture; Horizontal part of palatine bone; Greater palatine foramen; Interpalatine suture; Lesser palatine foramina

Figures 18.11/18.12

In the embryo, development of the maxilla and palatine bones closes the palate along the sagittal midline of the body. A cleft palate results when this closure is incomplete. Conversely, a pronounced palatine raphe (an anterior/posterior ridge along the palate's intermaxillary and interpalatine midline sutures) may be a result of cranial crowding or narrowing of the palate.

To clarify, we aren't trying to release or differentiate the soft tissue or myofascia of the palate—we're waiting for a change in bony mobility. Although subtle, this tangible yielding of bony resilience indicates suture response and an increase of osseous adaptability. Although your touch is receptive, this isn't the light touch of craniosacral work. While skilled craniosacral work can be extraordinarily helpful for migraines, in this technique we use firm, tangible pressure, and wait for a small yet perceptible yielding. The pacing of your pressure is slow and steady. Imagine pushing a boat away from a dock (one of my favorite metaphors for this approach)—at first, there is no movement, but as you lean and wait, the boat yields and begins to drift. At the risk of mixing metaphors, another way to describe what we're feeling for might be the tactile "give" that a nearly ripe avocado would have.

A pronounced palatine raphe (a sagittal or anterior/posterior ridge along the palate's midline sutures, Figure 18.5) can sometimes be a result of cranial crowding or narrowing of the palate. If you encounter a sagittal ridge, use gentle but firm outward pressure on the palate, still without sliding, in order to encourage widening and lateral easing of the roof of the mouth.

A cleft palate could be thought of as the opposite—a palate with too much lateral space. In fetal development (Figures 18.11 and 18.12), the bones of a cleft palate never met and closed along the centerline. Anecdotally, I have worked with several clients whose cleft palates had been surgically repaired, and who also suffered from migraines. Keeping in mind our "decompression" metaphor, we can imagine that the closing of the previously too-open palate was accomplished in a way that didn't allow for normal palatine adaptability and mobility.

Why does mobilizing the bones of the palate so often reduce migraine pain? Perhaps it is through an effect on the trigeminal nerve, which branches into the greater palatine and nasopalatine nerves above and below the palate (Figure 18.13). Or perhaps the direct pressure is transmitted through the vertical fin of the vomer into the sphenoid bone and the cranial base (Figures 18.14 and 18.15), where the pituitary and hypothalamus are situated (both of which may play a role in the neuro-electrical "brainstorm" of a migraine). Since much of the venous drainage of the cranial vault occurs through foramina in this area, we may be helping decrease intracranial pressure by opening the vascular "drains" of the vault. Whatever the reason it works, I am confident that you and your migraine clients will come to value this technique.

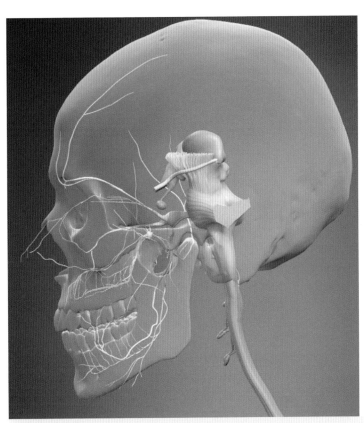
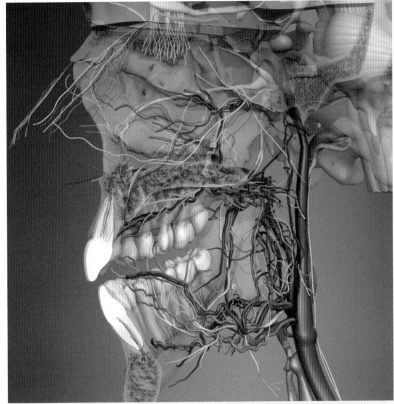

Figures 18.13/18.14

The trigeminal nerve and the brainstem, two of the neural structures implicated in both migraine and cluster headache pain. Our metaphorical goal of decompressing the cranial bones may give relief to migraines by relieving pressure on the trigeminal nerve branches. One of these, the greater palatine nerve (green) may be a key why work on the hard palate seems to often relieve migraine pain.

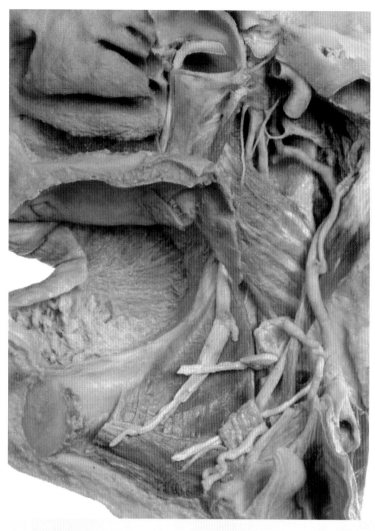

Figure 18.15

The trigeminal nerve's ganglia and maxillary nerve roots (green) in dissection.

And of course, it makes an ideal self-care method. Be sure to instruct your clients on how to perform it on themselves at the first sign of migraine.

Key points: Palate Technique

Indications include:
- Headaches, especially migraines and cluster headaches.
- Sinus issues.

Purpose
- Cranial decompression.
- Palatine adaptability.
- Symptomatic relief of headache pain.

Instructions
1. Use firm, static pressure to feel the shape and mobility or fixity of the bones that make up the palate.
2. Wait for a change in bony mobility, and/or change in headache pain.
3. In active headaches, solicit client feedback about placement, direction, and pressure that best addresses headache pain.
4. Encourage the client to breathe normally, as well as to relax the jaw, neck, and body.

External Acoustic Meatus Technique

Since our intention with migraines is to decompress the relationship between the cranial bones, the ears are convenient handles for applying traction directly to the temporal bones. The external part of the ear (or auricle) has firm fascial attachments to the surface of the temporal bone, and the ear canal (or acoustic meatus) passes deep into the temporal's petrous portion (Figure 18.16). The medial end of this petrous part cradles the trigeminal nerve where it emerges from the brainstem (the trigeminal nerve is likely involved in both migraines and

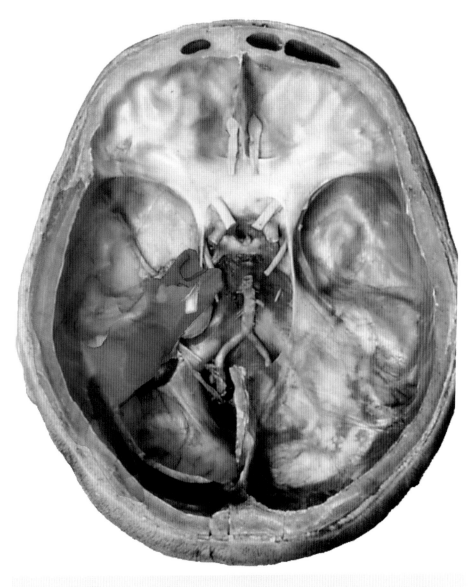

Figure 18.16

The ears are effective handles for applying traction to the temporal bone (superimposed in blue). The temporal's petrous portion (medial, darker violet) houses the acoustic meatus and the internal carotid artery, which supplies the cerebral hemispheres, eyes, and forehead. Its medial end cradles the trigeminal nerve (yellow).

cluster headaches). Aligned with the meatus and adjacent to it within the petrous portion of the temporal bone, are the carotid canal and the internal carotid artery. These supply blood to the cerebral hemispheres, eyes, and forehead—areas where migraineurs and cluster headache sufferers are often most affected.

Holding both ears' conchae (the inner cartilaginous bowl around the opening of the ear) as in Figure 18.17, apply sensitive but firm posterolateral traction. Use the ear canal to feel or imagine deep into the cranium. Ask your client about how much traction is comfortable; pull steadily, and wait for at least a few breaths. Try traction in slightly different directions, and stay in close verbal communication about which variations most affect the headache's pain. Sometimes the smallest adjustments to angle, grip, and pull make a large difference to your client's experience.

Ask your client to let you know if your traction seems to relate to their headache pain at all. Once you've found an angle that feels relevant to your client, simply hold the traction, imagining or feeling how the ear canals might actually connect with one another at a place a little anterior of the center of the head (which in one sense, they do, via their connective tissue linkages to the internal acoustic meatus and the cranial tentorium). Repeat this simple but profound release in a slightly different direction. Alternatively, you can grasp the tragus (the small external projection anterior to the opening of the ear canal), or the earlobes, to feel into different parts of the ear canal. As with palate work, be patient and thorough, staying in constant verbal communication with your client to get the angle and amount of traction just right.

Freeing the temporal bones in this way can relieve both migraines and musculoskeletal headaches. Musculoskeletal headaches respond especially well when you add active movement of the eyes and jaw (Figure 18.17) to extend the effects into these structures.

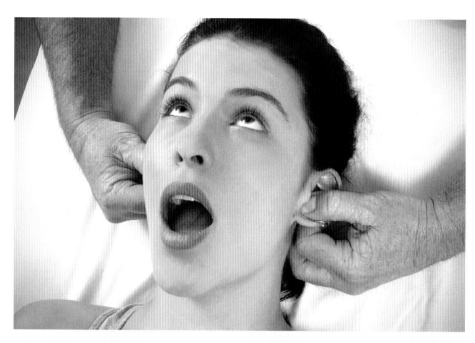

Figure 18.17

In the External Acoustic Meatus Technique, use firm but gentle posterolateral traction on the external ear to feel deeply into the fascial and osseous connections within the cranium. Active movement of the eyes and jaw can augment and broaden this technique's effects.

Key points: External Acoustic Meatus Technique

Indications include:
- Headaches, both musculoskeletal and neurovascular.
- TMJD; eyestrain; facial tension or pain.

Purpose
- Cranial decompression via mobilization of the temporal bones.

Instructions
- Apply gentle but firm traction to the external acoustic meatus, conchae, or tragus of the ears, at different angles
- Feel or imagine deep into the fascial, osseous, and nervous connections within the head
- Solicit client feedback about placement, direction, and pressure that best addresses headache or other pain

Movements
- Utilize the client's active eye, jaw, and facial movements

Contraindications
- Probably contraindicated after cosmetic surgery involving the ear region.

Do good work

It is always a good idea to have your client check with his or her physician in the case of recurring, severe, or persistent headaches, even if you are able to relieve the pain with the methods described here. In most cases, headaches are uncomfortable but benign; however, they can be a sign of other problems and a medical doctor should rule these out, just to be safe.

Although hands-on work can provide very welcome relief for migraine and cluster headache suffers, it is wise to be optimistically balanced in our expectations about completely "curing" migraines. Migraines can be complicated, and sometimes seem to have multiple causes. Although I have had very good luck at relieving acute migraine pain in my practice (with an unscientific estimate of perhaps 90 percent reporting at least some improvement), it is harder to estimate the percentage of clients who have an ongoing and lasting improvement in migraine frequency or intensity, (though stories of improvement in those areas are also common). Regularity seems to be an important key: the two studies already cited of migraine improvement after hands-on work (Hernandez-Reif 1998 and Lawler 2006) both employed regular, repeated sessions.

Whether or not we permanently "cure" our clients' vascular headaches, or simply provide them with welcome symptomatic relief, I'm confident you'll find that hands-on work can play an extremely useful role in managing the pain of migraines, and in preventing the stress and myofascial strain that can trigger them.

References

[1] Dodick, D.W. and Gargus, J.J. (2008) Why migraines strike: Biologists are finally unraveling the medical mysteries of migraine, from aura to pain. *Scientific American*. August. p. 56–63.

[2] Stovner, L.J., Zwart, J.A., Hagen, K., Terwindt, G.M., and Pascual, J. (2006) Epidemiology of headache in Europe. *European Journal of Neurology*. 13(4) p. 333–345.

[3] Gervil, M., Ulrich, V., Kaprio, J., Olesen, J., and Russell, M.B. (1999) The relative role of genetic and environmental factors in migraine without aura. *Neurology*. 53(5) p. 995–999.

[4] Kantor, D. (2006) Migraine. *MedlinePlus Medical Encyclopedia*. http://www.nlm.nih.gov/medlineplus/ency/article/000709.htm. [Accessed December 2015]

[5] Dodick, D.W. and Gargus, J.J. ibid.

[6] Alexandre, F., DaSilva, C.G., Snyder, J., and Hadjikhani, N. (2007) Thickening in the somatosensory cortex of patients with migraine. *Neurology*. 69. p. 1990–1995.

[7] Matharu, M. and Goadsby, P. (2001) Cluster headache: Update on a common neurological problem. *Practical Neurology 1*. p. 42–49.

[8] Fischera, M., Marziniak, I., Gralow, S., and Evers, S. (2008) The incidence and prevalence of cluster headache: A meta-analysis of population-based studies. *Cephalalgia*. 28(6). p. 614–618.

[9] Weaver-Agostoni, J. (2013) Cluster headache. *American Family Physician*. (Review) 88(2). p. 122–128.

[10] Two studies that show beneficial effects of hands-on work with migraine sufferers are: Hernandez-Reif, M. et al. (1998) Migraine headaches are reduced by massage therapy. *International Journal of Neuroscience*. 96. p. 1–11; and Lawler, S.P. and Cameron, L.D. (2006) A randomized, controlled trial of massage therapy as a treatment for migraine. *Annals of Behavioral Medicine*. 32. p. 50–59.

[11] Hannan, K. (2005) Orthodontic braces and migraine headache: Prevalence of migraine headache in females aged 12–18 years with and without orthodontic braces. *International Journal of Osteopathic Medicine* 8(4). p. 146–151.

Picture credits

Study Guide

Migraines

1 The text says that migraines are currently thought to be primarily a:

a myofascial disorder
b vascular disorder
c nervous system disorder
d immune system disorder

2 When it is present, at what stage does vasodilation occur in migraine headaches, according to the chapter?

a before
b after
c during
d vasodilation is no longer thought to be associated with migraines

3 Since many migraines are also commingled (mixed type), the text says it can be useful to begin working with a migraine client by addressing:

a bony mobility restrictions
b myofascial tension
c jaw range of motion limitations
d any painful areas

4 In the Palate Technique, the practitioner is primarily feeling for a change in:

a muscular tension
b myofascial differentiation
c proprioceptive refinement
d bony mobility

5 The External Acoustic Meatus Technique suggests beginning with traction in which direction?

a anterolateral
b lateral
c posterolateral
d posterior

For Answer Keys, visit www.Advanced-Trainings.com

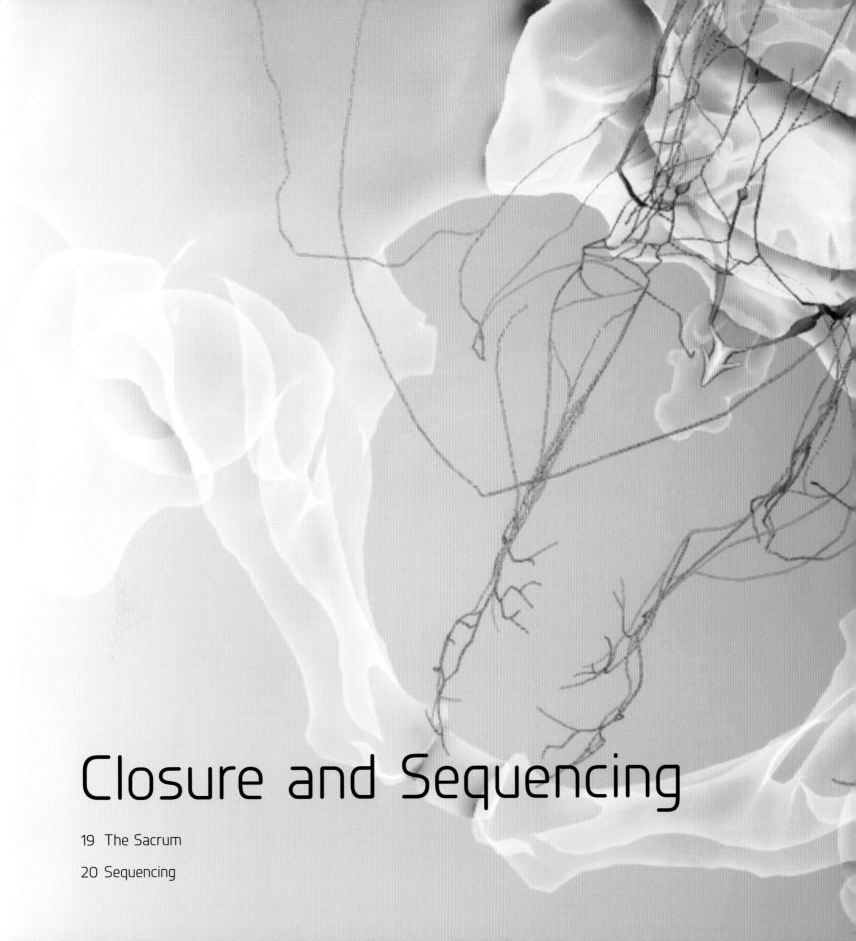

Closure and Sequencing

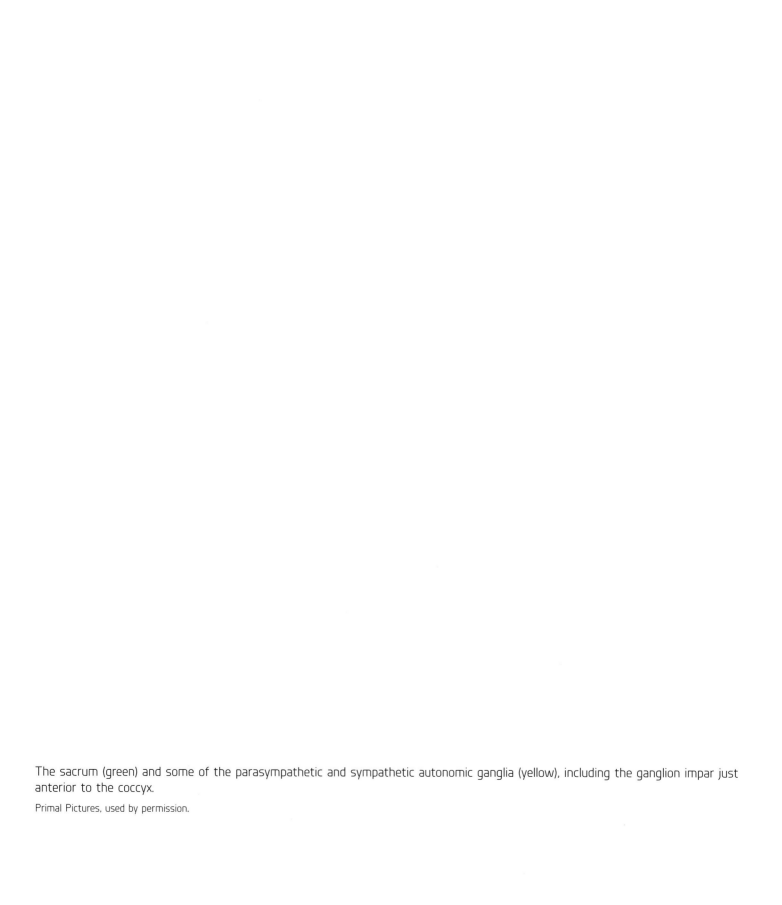

The sacrum (green) and some of the parasympathetic and sympathetic autonomic ganglia (yellow), including the ganglion impar just anterior to the coccyx.

The Sacrum

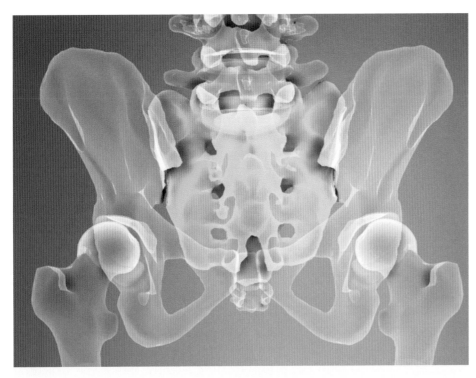

Figure 19.1

The sacrum (green) has special significance in many manual therapy methods.

The English word "sacrum" is a shortened form of the Latin *os sacrum* or "sacred bone." Prior to the mid 1700s, this bone was called *holy bone* in both English (1) and German (*heiliges bein*), where it is now referred to as the *Kreuzbein* (or "cross" bone) (2). The "sacred" or "holy" connotations of this bone's name are mysterious and speculative. Theories include the cross-shaped appearance of this bone in some animals; its supposed role in animal sacrificial rites, due to its proximity to reproductive organs; and its being the last bone to survive cremation in a sacrificial pyre (3). Since the original Greek root can be translated as either "sacred" or "strong," others conjecture that the Latin "sacred bone" was simply a mistranslation of "strongest bone;" (4) which is interesting to us since the sacrum, as the largest vertebral structure bears the weight of the entire spine.

Word origins aside, the sacrum (Figure 19.1) has a unique significance in many manual therapies. Osteopathic manipulation places special importance on sacral dynamics (5), and of course it figures prominently in the craniosacral approach that traces its roots to osteopathy. Structural bodywork emphasizes the sacrum's role in weight transfer from the upper body to the supporting lower limbs, and its function in mediating the movements between the left and right ilia and legs.

Autonomically, the sacral region is significant for its high concentration of parasympathetic nerve ganglia involved in visceral function (the "old vagal" branch), responsible for both deep relaxation, and for primitive biological responses to trauma (6). It is also the site of the ganglion impar, the single unpaired ganglion at the convergence of the left and right sympathetic trunks just anterior to the sacrum's juncture with the

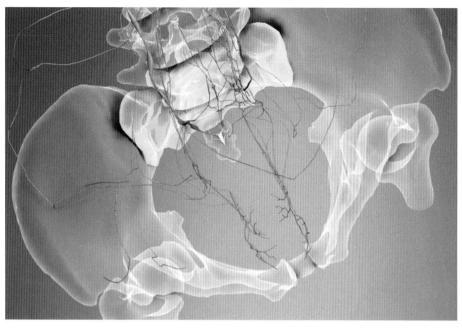

Figure 19.2

The concentrations of fine parasympathetic nerves and rounded ganglia near the sacrum may help explain the calming and quieting nature of sacral work. The ganglion impar is at the caudal convergence of the larger left and right sympathetic trunks, just anterior to the sacrum's juncture with the coccyx.

coccyx (Figure 19.2) which in yogic philosophy is the site of *muladhara chakra* where the *ida* and the *pingala* (the left and right *nadis* or energetic channels of the body) meet and are united (7).

Sacral shape varies greatly from person to person. In men, the sacrum is generally larger and more evenly curved throughout its shape. In women, the smaller and wider sacrum tends to be flatter in its superior part, but more concave in its inferior part than men's, with a sharper mid-sacral angle where these two parts meet. The sacrum, which initially forms as four to six separate vertebrae, has a relatively slow process of ossification. Children's sacral vertebrae remain completely separate until late-adolescence and do not fuse completely until around 30 years of age (8).

The pelvic lift

Ida Rolf PhD, the originator of Rolfing structural integration, finished most of her sessions with a "pelvic lift" maneuver, most likely inspired by her study with osteopath Amy Cochrane in the 1940s (9). More recently, author and structural integration teacher Thomas Myers described Ida Rolf's technique this way:

"In the pelvic lift, the client, supine with her knees up, rolls her pelvis up from the tailbone until the lumbars are off the table. The therapist slides a hand, palm up, under the lumbars, stretching and easing tissue along the posterior of the lumbars and sacrum as the client brings the pelvis slowly, segment by segment, back down to rest onto the practitioner's hand…

Hook your fingertips (by flexing your fingers) into the tissue on either side of the spine and draw downward toward the tailbone…be sure that your pull is straight toward the client's heels, not in a curve." (10).

What was the purpose of Rolf's pelvic lift? There were many. Myers quotes an archival list of 18 "Possible Pelvic-Lift Objectives" (attributed to the late Stacy Mills, one of Ida Rolf's first instructors, whom I also had the honor to study with in the mid-1980s) (11):

1. Disengage sacrum from L5.
2. Disengage L5 from L4.
3. Disengage L4 from L3, etc.
4. Engage the hinging of the sacrum below lumbars.
5. Engage the lumbo-dorsal hinge or thoracolumbar junction.
6. Lengthen and hydrate lumbar intervertebral discs.
7. Teach lumbars to fall back from lordosis.
8. Lengthen the thoracolumbar fascia.
9. Lengthen and ease sacral fascia.
10. De-rotate the lumbar column or specific vertebrae.
11. De-rotate an ilium, balance the two hip bones.
12. De-rotate the sacrum.
13. Ease or straighten coccyx.
14. Create ease at the SI joint.
15. Balance the craniosacral rhythm via the sacrum.
16. Ground client—stimulate parasympathetic autonomic tone.
17. Release or stimulate pelvic floor.
18. Horizontalize (find neutral position for) the pelvis.

The pelvic lift was Rolf's go-to technique when clients were agitated or unsettled. "A pelvic lift is always in order in an emergency," Rolf said, (12) and this observation was later borne out in some of the first formal research on Rolfing structural integration, which showed a persistent increase in vagal tone (a measure of parasympathetic activity) after receiving a pelvic lift (13).

Floating Sacrum Technique

As an alternative to the direct-traction technique described above, we often close our *Advanced Myofascial Techniques* sequences with a less directive, listening-based version of this sacral technique. A lighter, more receptive approach helps end a session on a quiet note, since this subtler type of work can be deeply calming. And rather than using direct work to add more input, more information, or more manipulation from the outside-in, the receptive approach of this technique also gives the client's somatic awareness time to register his or her own internal bodily perceptions, from the inside-out.

Begin by making sure your client understands why you propose working in this potentially personal area. Once you have clear agreement, ask your client to lift the hips just high enough so that you can place your hand squarely and comfortably under the client's sacrum (Figures 19.3 and 19.4), as described for the pelvic lift (above). Your other hand can rest on the client's knees, abdomen, or elsewhere (Figures 19.5 and 19.6). Rather than immediately "hooking in" or applying traction to the sacrum as you would in the direct version, simply allow the sacrum to rest on your hand. Let the sacrum come to you, like a boat settling into the water. Be sure you are comfortable and easy in your own body; this will ensure your touch is as receptive as possible.

Rather than move the sacrum, feel for whatever movements it is already making. In most cases, the breath motion will be clearly palpable here; by waiting quietly and listening even more, you'll become aware of other small, slow motions of this bone. It's not uncommon to feel the slow longitudinal rocking of the sacrum within the pelvis (the craniosacral pulse), which is said to have both longer and shorter cycles. You may also feel other motions: slow drifting, dropping, swiveling, or side-to-side motions. Don't let your ideas of conventional physics or joint biomechanics limit what you feel. Likewise, resist the urge to exaggerate, resist, correct, or manipulate these sacral motions for now; simply follow whatever motions you feel, or think you feel. Supporting the sacrum in this way can be profoundly relaxing for your client and will often produce a much deeper experience than more pushing, pulling, massaging, or manipulating.

You'll know enough time has passed when you notice one or more of these things:

- A shift in your client's movement rhythms (typically a slowing down, or a moment of stillness).
- A sign of autonomic change (such as a twitch, deep breath, eye flicker, etc.)
- Your own sense of finality (though it's usually best not to use your own restlessness as the only guide to timing your techniques).
- Your next client is arriving, meaning that you're out of time.
- Remove your hand, either by having your client reverse the process of lifting the hips off the table or by using the traction described above to end with a sense of length in the lumbar spine, and be sure to allow your client time to savor and soak in the restful quiet that this gentle technique can engender.

Key points: Floating Sacrum Technique

Indications include:
- Session closure.
- Pelvic, SI, or low back pain or instability.
- Agitation, disquiet, sympathetic activation, etc.

Purpose
- Parasympathetic activation; relaxation; calming.
- Normalize or calm sacral mobility.

Instructions
After getting client agreement for working in this area:
1. Ask client to lift pelvis, and place your hand squarely under the sacrum.
2. Get comfortable; relax.
3. Let the sacrum settle in your soft, receptive hand.
4. Feel for and follow sacrum's subtle motions, without directing, exaggerating, or inhibiting. Wait for ANS response or mobility shift.

See video of the Sacrum Technique at www.a-t.tv/sc09

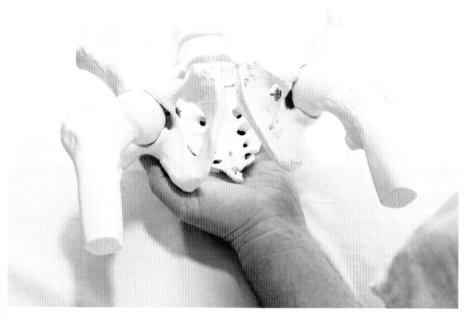

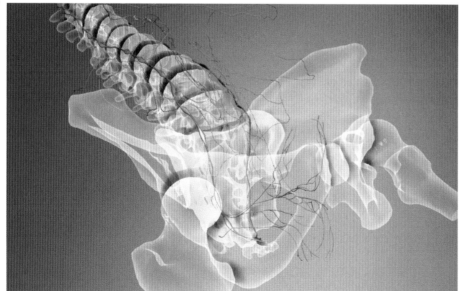

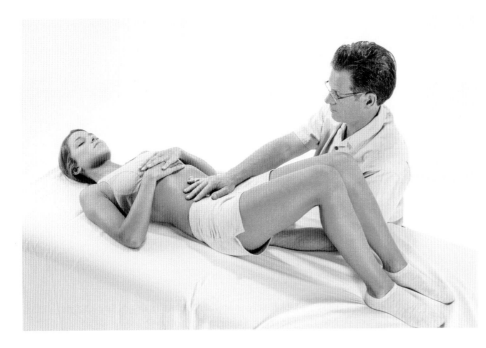

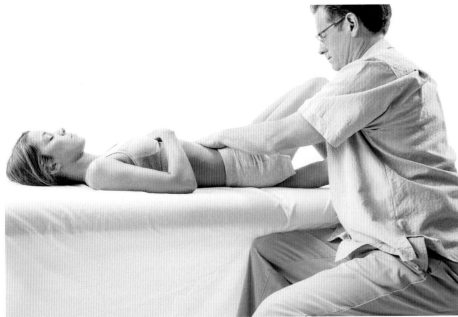

Figures 19.3/19.4/19.5/19.6

In the Floating Sacrum Technique, the practitioner's hand is centered under the client's sacrum. The upper hand can lightly rest on the abdomen as pictured, on the hipbones, or it can steady the client's knees. Once in position, the practitioner feels for and follows any subtle movements of the sacrum, such as breath rhythms, etc.

References

[1] Schreger, C.H.Th. (1805) Synonymia anatomica: Synonymik der anatomischen Nomenclatur. *Fürth: im Bureau für Literatur.*

[2] Grimm, J. and Grimm, W. *Deutsches Wörterbuch*. University of Trier. www.woerterbuchnetz.de/DWB/?sigle=DWB&mode=Vernetzung&-lemid=GK13393. [Accessed December 2015]

[3] Foster, F.P. and Ayres, W.C. (1891–1893) *An Illustrated Encyclopædic Medical Dictionary*. New York: D. Appleton and Company.

[4] Online Etymology Dictionary. www.etymonline.com/index.php?-term=sacrum. [Accessed December 2015]

[5] Chila, A.G. (2010) *Foundations of Osteopathic Medicine.* Lippincott Williams & Wilkins. p. 575.

[6] Porges, S.W. (2011) *The Polyvagal Theory: Neurophysiological Foundations of Emotions, Attachment, Communication, and Self-regulation.* New York: WW Norton.

[7] Upadhyaya, R. and Sharma, G. (2006) *Awake Kundalini.* Lotus Press. p. 99.

[8] Baker, J.B. et al. (2005) *The Osteology of Infants and Children.* Texas A & M University Press. p. 86.

[9] Bond, M. (2012) The pelvic lift: Theme and variations. www.healyourposture.com/wp-content/uploads/2012/02/pelvic-lift.pdf. [Accessed December 2015]

[10] Myers, T. (2013) The pelvic lift: A Rolf-approved session finisher. *Massage & Bodywork.* January/February.

[11] Myers, T. (2013) ibid.

[12] Bond, M. (2012) ibid.

[13] Cottingham, J.T. et al. (1988) Effects of soft tissue mobilization (Rolfing pelvic lift) on parasympathetic tone in two age groups. *Journal of American Physical Therapy Association.* 68(3). p. 352–356.

Picture credits

Study Guide

The Sacrum

1 **The text says sacral shape is:**

a flatter in women
b highly variable
c flatter in yogis
d more concave in men

2 **As described in the chapter, Ida Rolf's version of the pelvic lift included instructions to:**

a be sure to put the client's knees down if lumbar curve is flat
b be sure to unite the left and right nadis
c be sure your pull is not in a curve
d be sure to work from the outside-in

3 **Which of these most closely matches the meaning of the chapter's text, as it applies to the Floating Sacrum Technique?**

a Rather than move the sacrum, feel for whatever movements it is already making.
b Rather than just feel the sacrum, make sure it is moving already.
c Rather than move just the sacrum, move whatever is not moving already.
d Rather than follow the sacrum, feel for whatever movements it is not yet making.

4 **One purpose of the Floating Sacrum Technique is described as:**

a disengaging L4 from L3
b easing or straightening the coccyx
c helping things end on a quiet note
d to make sure the client understands why you're working in this potentially personal area

5 **Which of these choices is NOT specifically listed as a possible sign that the technique is complete:**

a your client twitches
b your client's spine lengthens caudally
c a shift in your client's movement rhythms
d your own sense of completion

For Answer Keys, visit www.Advanced-Trainings.com

Sequencing

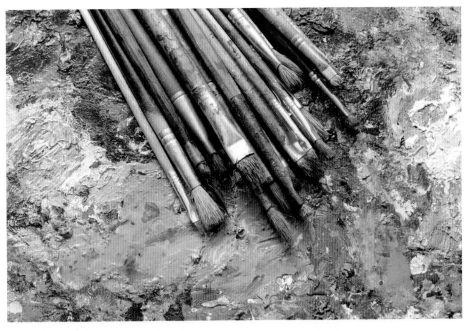

Figure 20.1

Techniques are tools, and are only as good as the skill with which they are used. Just as artists enter a new level of creativity and mastery once familiar with the tools and media of their craft, hands-on practitioners will be ready for more complex challenges, once the basics of the techniques have been learned.

The introduction to this book touched on how the techniques in these volumes can be incorporated one-by-one into your existing work and protocols, à la carte fashion, according to the indications and purposes listed in each technique's Key Points section, or, in any way you see fit. Although each of these techniques has been selected for their ability to stand on their own, they are part of a larger body of work, with its own logic and ways of viewing the body. As such, they will be even more effective when they are combined in progressions or sequences that support the overall aims of the client and practitioner.

Knowing *how* to do a technique is important, but perhaps even more important is knowing *when* to use it. This means not only knowing which technique addresses the particular condition or complaint at hand, but also, how to sequence the tools one chooses into a cohesive whole, with a beginning, middle, and end.

Many of the sections in this volume have been arranged in an order that can be used as a possible progression; the individual technique descriptions often include additional sequencing considerations. Further protocols and session sequences are available in the full-length videos and course notebooks of our in-person trainings (see Online Resources, page xix).

But, just as techniques are not all that is required for good body work, protocols also have their limits. At some point in their professional development, many practitioners look for ways to move beyond the scripts, recipes, and routines that originally helped them learn and apply their work. This is similar to how an artist, once familiar with the tools, media, and practices of the craft, enters a new level of mastery and creativity (Figure 20.1); or how a craftsman is ready

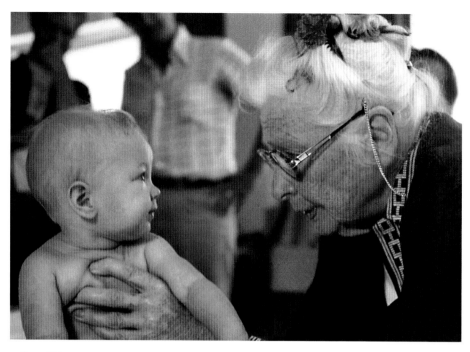

Figure 20.2

Dr. Ida P. Rolf, the originator of Rolfing® Structural Integration.

for new and more complex challenges, once the basics of the trade have been mastered.

As with any other craft or discipline, knowing when to apply a particular hands-on tool comes with experience and through getting to know the applications, effects, and limitations of the techniques. So, a certain amount of knowledge about effective sequencing comes simply by practicing and employing the techniques themselves.

It is also true that techniques don't exist in isolation. Techniques are woven together within a larger context that includes not only the other techniques they are combined with, but also the setting, scope, aims, or style that the work happens within. As this book is written for practitioners practicing in diverse settings, the sequencing and application of the techniques can vary greatly. There are, however, a few general principles that can guide your technique selection and sequencing.

Preparation, differentiation, and integration

Dr. Ida P. Rolf (Figure 20.2), the originator of Rolfing® Structural Integration, taught the sequencing of her work via a recipe of ten basic sessions that progressively addressed the body in its entirety (1). The logic of her original ten-session sequence has been analyzed, re-interpreted, and hotly debated amongst the various schools that continue her structural integration lineage. However, one of the most fundamental ways her original sequence can be understood is as a three-phase progression of *preparation* (the theme of the first three sessions in her series), *differentiation* (sessions four through seven), and *integration* (the final three sessions of her series).[1]

Without trying to replicate the specifics of Dr. Rolf's recipe, we adapt the general principles of preparation, differentiation, and integration

1 Even though we draw inspiration from this fundamental sequencing in our Advanced Myofascial Techniques work (and even though many Rolfers and structural integration practitioners are amongst our faculty and alumni of our in-person trainings), I should clarify that this work is not Rolfing® (which is trademarked by the Rolf Institute of Structural Integration®) or structural integration per se, because we are focusing on techniques to address specific conditions, rather than on integration of the entire body in the field of gravity, which is the aim of structural integration.

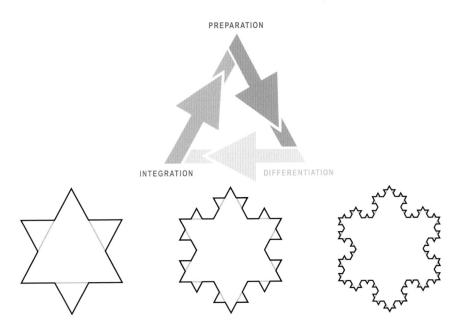

Figure 20.3

Preparation, Differentiation, and Integration as a repeating cycle that applies a single technique (large triangle) as well as to a session or series (smaller triangles), each of which is composed of smaller versions of the same beginning-middle-end cycle.

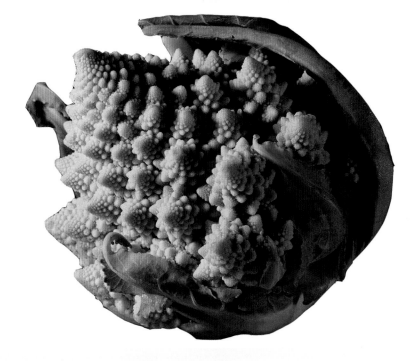

Figure 20.4

The self-similarity of Romanesco broccoli is one of the many examples from nature that illustrates how smaller units (e.g., techniques) make up similarly patterned larger units (sessions), which in turn make up the whole (a series of sessions).

in our myofascial approach. This three-phase progression can be applied to all scales and levels of the work, from an individual technique, to a session, to a series of sessions (Figure 20.3). This micro/macro repetition can be compared to a self-similar fractal-like design, where the same patterns are visible at all scales of magnification (Figure 20.4). Each technique needs preparation; a working phase (most often in this work, this involves differentiating one structure from another); and integration with the rest of the body, as well as the rest of the session. This same beginning-middle-end rhythm applies to the session as a whole, where the first techniques will be preparatory, and the last, integrative. It also applies to a series of sessions over time, where the effectiveness of the middle and ending sessions depend on the extent of preparation done in earlier sessions; and the degree of lasting change produced hinges on the integration that happens toward the end of the series. Let's look at each of these three phases in turn.

The many meanings of preparation

Preparation is defined as "the action or process of making ready" (2). Although preparation for hands-on work needs to include the physical aspects of "making ready" (such as relaxing excessive muscle tone, "warming up" or mobilizing superficial layers before working deeper structures, etc.), these physical considerations are only part of the picture.

Preparation as "making ready" begs the question, "ready for *what*?" As practitioners, we need to know our context and aim, in order to know how to prepare for them. In fact, one of the most important (and most overlooked) parts of the preparation phase is gaining clarity about the purpose and goals of the work itself—the client's reasons for seeking work and their hoped-for results; one's own goals, priorities, and aims as a practitioner; and most importantly, how these

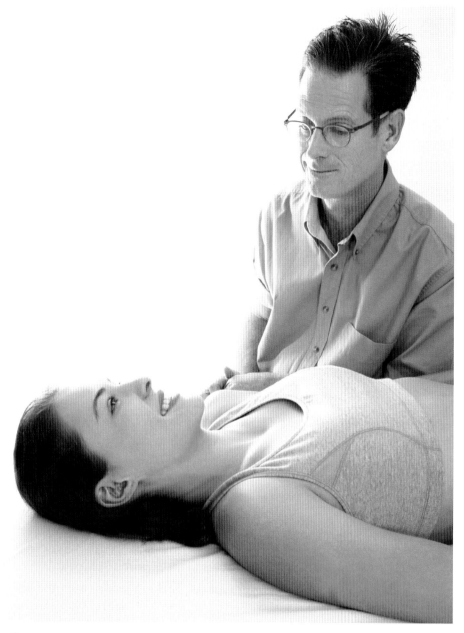

Figure 20.5

Taking time to ask, listen, and clarify what the client wants is indispensable verbal preparation for hands-on work.

two (the client's and the practitioner's priorities) intersect, or diverge. Many manual therapists are most comfortable working non-verbally, at what Dr. Rolf called "the silent level of the flesh" (3), and are often keen to get to work with their hands. Taking time to ask, listen, and clarify what the client wants from the work, and then exploring and discussing how this matches what you think you can deliver, is indispensable preparation for your hands-on work together (Figure 20.5).

The above considerations are small examples of what could be termed a "biopsychosocial" approach (4), which describes a whole-person, body-mind, context-dependent perspective on pain and symptoms. More and more conditions previously thought of as primarily physical complaints (such as TMJD, discussed in Chapters 14–16), are now seen as largely biopsychosocial phenomena, where the physical symptoms are only the most obvious aspects of a more complex, interdependent interplay of structure and function, and also of emotions, perceptions, beliefs, lifestyle, habits, social factors, and more (5).

In our *preparation* phase, we reverse the ordering of "biopsychosocial" so that it becomes "socio-psycho-bio:" before we can be maximally effectual in our biological or physical goals, the social aspects of the working relationship need to be established. This "social" level incudes all of the interpersonal interactions that enable the physical work to be effective: building rapport and trust; as well as establishing the tone, boundaries, and style of the therapeutic coalition. Therapeutic effectiveness in both physical medicine and in other fields has been shown to correlate with the strength of the practitioner-patient alliance (6). (Later, we'll see how "compliance," or the client's willingness to follow the practitioner's suggestions between sessions, depends on this social rapport as well.)

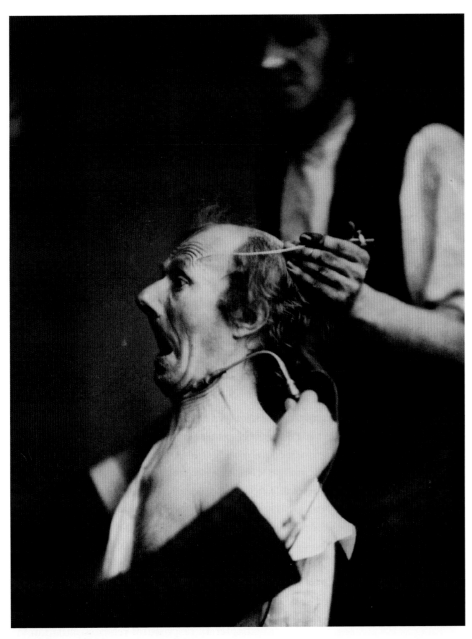

Figure 20.6

Sympathetic "fight or flight" states, like those accompanying anxiety, fear, unresolved trauma, or pain, can be aggravated by hands-on work that is too direct, too fast, or too deep. Preparation may involve calming and modulating these responses before proceeding with direct structural work. The photograph shows French neurologist Guillaume Duchenne de Boulogne, 1801–1875, investigating the relationship between electrostimulus of facial muscles and the expression of various emotions, including fear, in a patient suffering from an anesthetic condition of the face.

These interpersonal, social-level aspects dovetail with the inner, intra-personal, psychological considerations of our "socio-psycho-bio" progression. These intra-personal aspects include the client's mood, receptivity, optimism, or pessimism; their largely unconscious assessment of the situation's safety or risk; as well as their conceptualizations, stories, and ideas about their presenting issues. Chronic symptoms, especially those that haven't responded well to other interventions, can be laden with difficult feelings (depression, hopelessness, etc.), self-perpetuating fears and limitations (such as the fear of movement), or fixed attitudes and belief structures. Our scope of practice as manual therapists doesn't typically include direct psychological work per se, which requires a different kind of training, sensitivity, and therapeutic paradigm. But we can have enormous influence on our client's perspective and mindset about their symptoms through our own approach and attitude. *Preparation* in this realm can mean fostering an emotional ambience that makes the desired change more likely, largely by cultivating those attitudes in ourselves, and in our client interactions. Some of these states include curiosity, respect, warmth, patience, gentleness, humor, etc.

A related aspect of preparation has to do with the client's state of autonomic nervous system (ANS) arousal (Figure 20.6). When there is a high level of sympathetic (fight or flight) activation, addressing this state often takes precedence over structural goals. Whether this ANS arousal is related to unresolved traumatic responses, chronic pain, anxiety, or the stresses of daily life, an on-alert, hyper-aroused, and hyper-sensitive state not only precludes learning and change, but can be aggravated by work that is too direct or deep. Fortunately, there are very effective hands-on and proprioceptive approaches to ANS

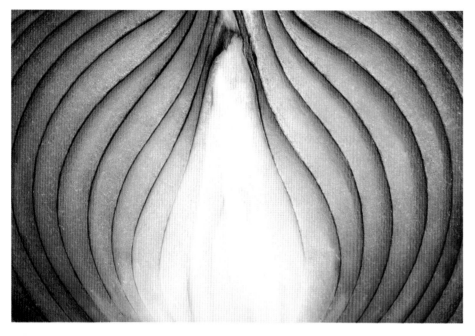

Figure 20.7
One method of preparation for deeper techniques involves first working the outer, most superficial layers of the body, which can be thought of being layered like an onion.

arousal, such as those discussed in Chapter 8, *The Vestibular System*, and Chapter 9, *Hot Whiplash*.

The psychological aspect of preparation could be defined within hands-on work as *fostering the internal conditions necessary for change to occur*. This would, of course, include readying oneself as a practitioner: becoming mentally, physically, and emotionally present, available, and primed for the work.

When we're ready for the hands-on portion of the work, preparation takes a more biological or physical meaning. Often, using the metaphor of body-as-onion (Figure 20.7), we start working with superficial layers of the body, in preparation for deeper work, such as in Chapter 11, The Superficial Cervical Fascia Technique. Another preparatory strategy we use (influenced by the work of Jan Sultan, one of Ida Rolf's original faculty) is to address the periphery of the body first (the appendicular extremities and girdles), before working with axial issues.

Our aims at this *preparation* stage include:

- Assessing and understanding the issues at hand (as in the Nod Test, Chapter 12, or the Lateral Pterygoid assessment, Chapter 15);
- Increasing tissue elasticity, hydration, and temperature (literally or metaphorically "warming up" the tissues, as in the Mother Cat Technique, Chapter 13); and
- Reducing motor tonus through autonomic calming (for example, the Vestibular Orienting Technique in Chapter 8), heightened proprioception (such as in the Vertebral Mobility Technique in Chapter 1), or postural reflex stimulation via Golgi tendon organ responses (as in the Posterior Digastrics Technique in Chapter 14).

Differentiation

The middle phase of our three-step sequencing cycle is *differentiation*, or the process of clarifying the distinctions between one thing and

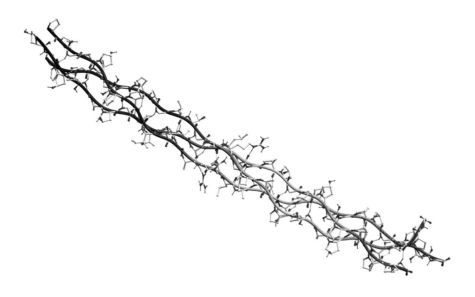

Figure 20.8

Collagen molecules, the most abundant fibrous component of most kinds of fascia, lend stiffness to myofascia by being chemically cross-linked with other collagen molecules.

another. In the body, we increase differentiation whenever we work to separate or mobilize one structure in relation to adjacent structures. Techniques such as the Intercostal Space Technique (Chapter 7) or the Cervical Translation Technique (Chapter 10) work to differentiate and mobilize bony structures (respectively, the individual ribs and the cervical vertebrae). Other techniques, such as the Thoracolumbar Fascia Technique (Chapter 1) or the Cervical Core/Sleeve Technique (Chapter 10), focus on differentiation of fascial layers. This usually means increasing the glide (or shear) between fascial layers, so that their movement is easier, freer, and less restricted.

At the microscopic level, our work, like comparable direct myofascial methods, is likely altering the quality and amount of hyaluronic acid (or hyaluronan), a slippery, large-molecule carbohydrate polymer found in abundance (amongst other places) between layers of fascia. Related to its function as a lubricating substance, hyaluronan plays a suspected role in myofascial pain (7). The pressure and shear of direct manual work also likely changes the enzymatic cross-linking between collagen molecules (Figure 20.8), helping these fibers move more freely against one another (8) and so decrease the potential stiffness and binding that is the downside of fascia's continuity.[2]

Differentiation applies not only to physical freedom and mobility, such as in the examples above, but also to proprioception and movement coordination. Many of our active-movement techniques (such as the two Psoas techniques in Chapter 5) help refine clients' initiation and control of finer movements. Hands-on work can also help increase the brain's ability to distinguish between different parts of the body, enhancing sensation, movement coordination, balance, and posture (Figure 20.9). Skilled touch can also help with the more severe loss

2 Fascia's unique properties of continuity, plasticity, and sensitivity, and the ways these qualities inform our work, are discussed in detail in the first two chapters of Volume 1.

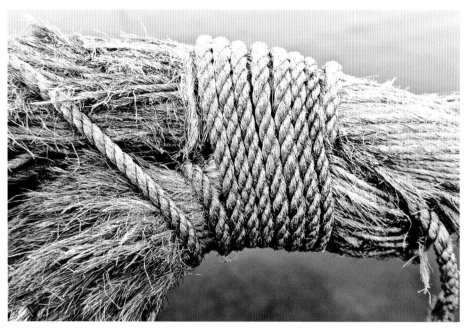

Figure 20.9

Fascia comes from the Latin word for band, bundle, or binding. This rope bundle metaphorically illustrates how undifferentiated fascia can bind and restrict bodily movement and functioning.

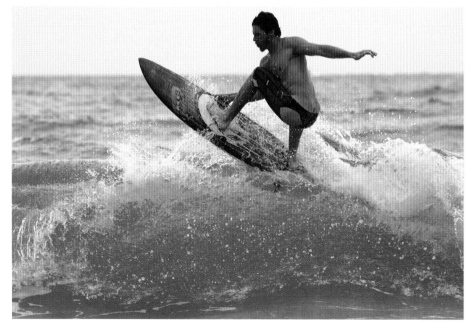

Figure 20.10

Differentiation of physical structures, and of their proprioceptive perceptions, enhances movement coordination, posture, balance, and overall body awareness.

of proprioceptive differentiation in the somatosensory "smudging" of chronic pain (9), allodynia (10) (pain related to sensations normally not painful), and in the somatic dissociation of unresolved trauma (11).

In this approach, *differentiation* is often our main method of improving both physical functioning (e.g., movement) and sensory phenomena (such as pain) (Figure 20.10). Increased functional and perceptual differentiation allows greater freedom of movement, more accurate body awareness, refined balance and coordination, and enhanced structural adaptability.

Integration

The term "integration" has come to mean many different things. Its Latin root, *integrāre*, means to renew or restore. In psychology, *integration* refers to the coordination of processes in the nervous system, including diverse sensory information and motor impulses, as in *visuomotor integration*. In the specialized vernacular of Rolfing and other forms of structural integration, *integration* is a very nuanced term that can imply balance, fullness, completion, alignment, ease, and more.

In its dictionary meaning, "integration" signifies the process of combining or uniting multiple things so they become a single whole. In our trainings, we use it mainly in this sense: the integration phase of our work reminds the body that it is not simply differentiated parts, but an irreducible, undivided whole.

In the earlier preparation phase of our three-part sequencing cycle, we reversed the ordering of "biopsychosocial," emphasizing the establishment of helpful inter- and intra-personal contexts before working on the biological level. In the final integration phase, we return to the original ordering of "biopsychosocial:" it is useful to think of addressing the biological or physical aspects of integration first; then the psychological or inner side of the work; and finally, the social, or interactive aspects of taking the work out into one's life (event though in practice, all these functions probably need to be addressed together, rather than sequentially).

The physical or biological aspects of integration and closure typically include attention to overall balance and territorial completeness. Does the work feel even and complete enough to the client to comfortably end the session? Different manual therapy modalities will accomplish this in different ways. Massage therapists, who are sometimes taught to work the entire body in every session, or at least both sides of the body, can often advance their skill by learning to achieve a sense of completeness even when working asymmetrically. On the other hand, physical therapists or physiotherapists, who typically receive a very detailed education about individual conditions and parts, can often round out their approach by looking for larger, unexpected connections in the body as a part of balancing and completing their work.

One of the best techniques for achieving this sense of balance is to simply ask the client or patient about their felt sense of completeness before your time with them is over. This psycho- (internal experience) social (interpersonal) approach might be phrased as, "If you check in with your body, is there something else that would help you feel complete for now?" This is very different than, "Is your pain still there?" which is a question that potentially opens a new chapter, rather than closing the existing one.

Dr. Rolf ended most of her sessions with neck work (similar to our Cervical Core/Sleeve Technique, Chapter 10) and a pelvic lift (a more direct version of the Sacrum Technique, Chapter 19). Her consistent use of this two-part closing ritual (probably rooted in osteopathic approaches) has been explained in many different ways. Interpretations include ensuring adaptability at each end of the spine to prevent later discomfort; working the midline of the body after working each side; and quieting the nervous system by working the two main areas of parasympathetic concentration (the cranial and caudal ends of the spine). All of these are worthy aims, but whatever the explanation, and even though we have diverged in many ways from Rolf's original protocols, we typically honor this closing custom, performing some sort of neck and sacrum work at the end of our Advanced Myofascial Techniques session sequences.

At the end of a technique, session, or series, our intention switches from separating, freeing, and differentiating distinct parts, to emphasizing larger connections and relationships between those parts. Sometimes this is done physically, with direct touch or pressure (as in the Core Point Technique in Volume 1, Chapter 1). At other times, we utilize the client's inner experience (the middle part of "biopsychosocial"), through guided awareness and sensory exploration (for example, the Psoas techniques in Chapter 5, or the Breath Motility Technique in Chapter 9).

Typically, in the *integration* phase of a technique or session, our touch style becomes receptive, rather than active; listening and sensing, rather than differentiating or manipulating. This allows the client's own proprioceptive awareness to come to the fore, and builds in a resting phase after more active work.

The final "social" aspect of our integration phase refers to the client's ability to integrate the awareness and changes from the session or series, into actual interactions and daily life. This is a social-level consideration in at least two ways:

1. New somatic patterns and awareness can be more challenging to recall and revisit when in relationship with other people and things, than they are in the quiet, internal focus of the practice room. Our interactions with clients as they rise, reschedule, and depart are valuable opportunities to tactfully invite clients

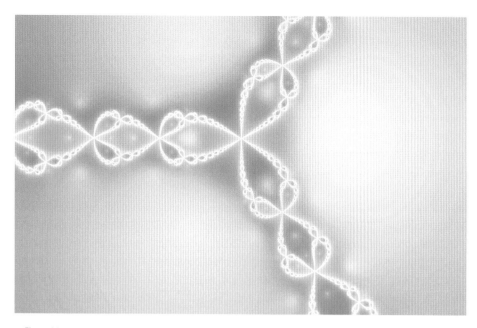

Figure 20.11

The micro/macro repetition of the Preparation, Differentiation, and Integration cycle can be compared to the self-similar design of the 3-element Julia set fractal, where similarly shaped patterns (such as the tricolored teardrop) are visible at all scales of magnification.

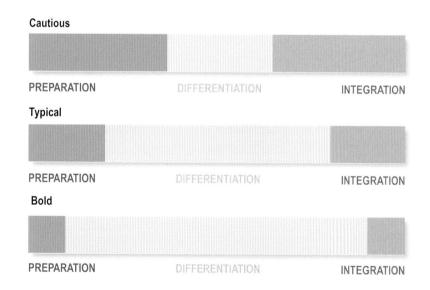

Cautious

| PREPARATION | DIFFERENTIATION | INTEGRATION |

Typical

| PREPARATION | DIFFERENTIATION | INTEGRATION |

Bold

| PREPARATION | DIFFERENTIATION | INTEGRATION |

Figure 20.12

The proportion of time, techniques, or sessions spent in each phase of the Preparation/Differentiation/Integration cycle can be varied according the condition being addressed. Top: a very cautious approach, such as would be appropriate for complex or less predictable conditions, such as hot whiplash or intervertebral disc issues. Bottom: a bold, direct approach with minimal preparation can be effective with stubborn conditions, especially when rapport and familiarity with the client's post-session responses have already been established.

to continue the proprioceptive awareness that will help carry the practice-room experience out into their lives.

2. Many modalities include client "homework," such as awareness practices or physical exercises, to help integrate and continue the work of the session. While such homework is undoubtedly useful (even indispensible in some cases), clients are notoriously inconsistent in their follow-through and between-session practice. How does this relate to the social level of our bio-psycho-social progression? Factors affecting "compliance" (the client or patient's adherence to the practitioner's homework, prescriptions, or recommendations) have been extensively studied in both physical and behavioral medicine. Influences such as client knowledge about their condition, social support (12) (family or social group awareness of practitioner recommendations), and client/practitioner rapport (13) all significantly increase the likelihood that homework recommendations will actually be followed. While most manual therapy practitioners probably see social support as being outside their typical scope of practice or sphere of influence, simply suggesting that clients share impressions of their sessions, or teach their homework to a friend, spouse, or family member, can help leverage the powerful social-support effect, and is very likely to increase the integration of the hands-on work into the client's habits and daily life.

How much is enough?

The sequence of preparation-differentiation-integration can provide a simple but useful conceptual framework for strategizing your sessions. As mentioned, this cycle applies in a fractal, self-similar fashion (Figure 20.11) to all levels of the work, from an individual technique (which needs to be eased into, sustained, and eased out of); to a single session (which optimally includes techniques that accomplish each

Technique	Preparation	Differentiation	Integration
Vertebral Mobility Technique	P	**D**	I
Iliac Crest Technique	P	D	
Thoracolumbar Fascia Technique	P	**D**	
Iliolumbar Ligament Technique		D	
12th Rib Technique		D	
Mesentery Technique	P	D	I
Psoas Technique (Supine)		D	I
Psoas Technique (Lateral)		D	I
Coastal Arch/Diaphragm Technique		D	
Erector Technique	P	**D**	I
Costovertebral Joint Technique		D	
Intercostal Space Technique		D	
Vestibular Orienting Technique	**P**		I
Breath Motility Technique	P	D	**I**
Cervical Core/Sleeve Technique	P	D	**I**
Lateral Cervical Translation Technique		D	I
Over the Edge Technique		D	
Cervical/Pectoralis Fascia Technique	P	**D**	
Nod Test	**P**		I

Technique	Preparation	Differentiation	Integration
Transversospinalis Technique	P	**D**	I
Cervical Wedge Technique		D	I
Anterior Scalene Technique		D	
Mother Cat Technique	P	D	**I**
TMJ Tracking	**P**		I
Masseter and Temporalis Technique	P	**D**	I
Anterior Digastric Technique		D	I
Posterior Digastric Technique		D	I
Masseter (Intraoral) Technique		D	
Medial Pterygoids		D	
Lateral Pterygoids		D	
Masseter (Intraoral) Technique		D	
Mandibular Fascia Technique			I
Galea Aponeurotica Technique	P	**D**	I
Nuchal Window Technique	P	D	**I**
External Acoustic Meatus Technique	**P**		I
Palate Technique		D	
Sacrum Technique	P		**I**

Table 20.1 Optimally, each session (as well as an entire series of sessions) is a progression of techniques that accomplish the preparation-differentiation-integration cycle. Table 20.1 lists possible usage of the techniques in this volume, with the most common function of a technique listed in bold type when a technique can serve more than one function.

of these three functions; see Table 20.1); and to a series of sessions, where the initial sessions are preparatory, followed by focused differentiation work addressing the chief concerns, and ending with sessions that emphasize the whole rather than the parts.

The proportion of time, techniques, or sessions you spend in each of these phases can be adjusted, depending on the stability, fragility, responsiveness, or stubbornness of the issues being addressed. In complex, unstable, or less-predictable conditions, such as spinal disc issues, hot whiplash, or symptomatic scoliosis, a very cautious approach (Figure 20.12) with proportionally more time spent in preparation and integration than with a typical progression gives you time to observe how your client responds to the work; and if necessary, to course-correct before aggravating the condition. In other cases, where the body or symptoms seem slow to show any response, a bolder, more direct approach might be appropriate. Even in slow-to-respond conditions, the results are usually greater when the preparation-phase functions of assessment, rapport, relaxation, and peripheral mobility have been thoroughly addressed.

Finally, whatever sequencing protocols you choose, the adage "less is more" seems to hold true. Whether it is from trying to give clients their money's worth, or inexperience with prioritization and time management, or fear of leaving something out, a common trait of beginning therapists is to do more than is necessary. The results can be overworking the client past the point of maximum benefit, dilution of the educational value of a few clear concepts for the client to incorporate, and practitioner burnout. There is almost always benefit in slowing down and spending more time with fewer techniques, than in rushing through as many as possible in the allotted time. On occasion, try "cooking" your sessions with just one or two spices, instead of using every seasoning in the cabinet. Or, let the sessions you compose have the spare beauty and spaciousness of a string quartet, rather than always going for the lushness of the full symphony orchestra. The effectiveness and satisfaction that both you and your client get from your work, depend less on how much you can fit in, and more on the art of leaving things out.

References

[1] Rolf, I.P. (1989) *Rolfing: Reestablishing the Natural Alignment and Structural Integration of the Human Body for Vitality and Well-Being*. Healing Arts Press.

[2] www.merriam-webster.com. http://www.merriam-webster.com/dictionary/preparation. [Accessed December 2015]

[3] Johnson, D.H. (1989) Presence. In: Carlson, R. and Shield, B. *Healers on Healing*. J.P. Tarcher. p. 133.

[4] Borrell-Carrió, F., Suchman, A.L., and Epstein, R.M. (2004) The biopsychosocial model 25 years later: Principles, practice, and scientific inquiry. *Annals of Family Medicine*. 2(6). p. 576–582.

[5] Scrivani, S.J., Keith, D.A., and Kaban, L.B. (2008) Temporomandibular disorders. *The New England Journal of Medicine*. 359. p. 2693–2705.

[6] Pinto, R.Z. et al. (2012) Patient-centred communication is associated with positive therapeutic alliance: A systematic review. *Journal of Physiotherapy*. 58(2). p. 77–87.

[7] Stecco, C., Stern, R., Porzionato, A., Macchi, V., Masiero S., Stecco A., and De Caro, R. (2011) Hyaluronan within fascia in the etiology of myofascial pain. *Surgical and Radiologic Anatomy*. 33(10). p. 891–896.

[8] Reiser, K., McCormick, R.J., and Rucker, R.B. (1992) Enzymatic and nonenzymatic cross-linking of collagen and elastin. *The FASEB Journal*. 6(7). p. 2439–2449.

[9] Butler, D.S. and Moseley, G.L. (2013) *Explain Pain*. 2nd ed. NOI Group.

[10] Allisona, G.T., Nagyb, B.M. and Hall, T. 2002. A randomized clinical trial of manual therapy for cervico-brachial pain syndrome: A pilot study. *Manual Therapy*. 7(2). p. 95–102.

[11] Scaer, R. (2014) *The Body Bears the Burden: Trauma, Dissociation, and Disease*. 3rd ed. Routledge. p. 166.

[12] DiMatteo, R.M. (2004) Social support and patient adherence to medical treatment: A meta-analysis. *Health Psychology*. 23(2). p. 207–218

[13] Howgego, M., Yellowlees, P., Owen, C., Meldrum, L., and Dark, F. (2003) The therapeutic alliance: The key to effective patient outcome? *Australian and New Zealand Journal of Psychiatry*. 37(2). p. 169–183.

Picture credits

Figures 20.1, 20.7, 20.8, 20.9, and 20.10 Thinkstock

Figure 20.2 courtesy Ron Thompson, used by permission.

Figures 20.3, 20.5, 20.12, 20.13, and 20.14 Advanced-Trainings.com. The three Koch snowflakes in Figure 20.3 are used under CC BY-SA 3.0.

Figure 20.4 Photographer: Jon Sullivan PDPhoto.org. Public domain image.

Figure 20.6 From Guillaume-Benjamin-Amand Duchenne de Boulogne, *Mécanisme de la physionomie humaine. ou, Analyse électro-physiologique de l'expression des passions des arts plastiques*. 1862. Public domain image.

Figure 20.11. The fractal Julia set (in white) for the rational function associated to Newton's method for f: z → z3−1. Coloring of Fatou set according to attractor (the roots of f). Public domain image, created by Georg-Johann Lay.

Study Guide

Sequencing

1 The Cervical Translation Technique is given here as an example of a technique that helps with:

a preparation
b differentiation
c integration
d cervical mobility

2 Which of these statements maintains the closest meaning to the way the same idea is phrased in the text?

a In order to be maximally effective towards our interpersonal goals, the client's physical goals must be addressed.
b In order to be maximally sensitive towards our clients' intra-personal goals, their physical goals need to be secondary.
c In order to be maximally effective towards our physical goals, the social aspects of the working relationship need to be established.
d In order to be maximally effective in the working relationship, the practitioner's therapeutic goals need to be primary.

3 Which of these is closest to the text? "The psychological aspect of preparation could be defined within hands-on work as…"

a "…fostering the interpersonal conditions necessary for change to occur."
b "…fostering the internal conditions necessary for change to occur."
c "…getting clear about clients' reasons for seeking work, and their hoped-for results."
d "…getting clear about the practitioner's therapeutic goals and hoped-for results."

4 "Reducing motor tonus through autonomic calming" is cited as an a goal typical of:

a preparation
b differentiation
c integration
d biopsychosociology

5 Which of these is NOT listed in the text as an interpretation of Ida Rolf's practice of working with the neck and pelvis at the end of her sessions?

a quieting the nervous system by working areas of parasympathetic concentration
b emphasizing the body's longitudinal axis in order encourage vertical alignment
c ensuring adaptability at each end of the spine to prevent later discomfort
d working the midline of the body after working each side

Index

Note: Page number followed by f and t indicates figure and table respectively.